Approaches to Improving the Quality of Life

Social Indicators Research Series

Volume 42

This new series aims to provide a public forum for single treatises and collections of papers on social indicators research that are too long to be published in our journal Social Indicators Research. Like the journal, the book series deals with statistical assessments of the quality of life from a broad perspective. It welcomes the research on a wide variety of substantive areas, including health, crime, housing, education, family life, leisure activities, transportation, mobility, economics, work, religion and environmental issues. These areas of research will focus on the impact of key issues such as health on the overall quality of life and vice versa. An international review board, consisting of Ruut Veenhoven, Joachim Vogel, Ed Diener, Torbjorn Moum, Mirjam A.G. Sprangers and Wolfgang Glatzer, will ensure the high quality of the series as a whole.

For futher volumes:
http://www.springer.com/series/6548

Abbott L. Ferriss

Approaches to Improving the Quality of Life

How to Enhance the Quality of Life

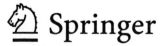 Springer

Prof. Abbott L. Ferriss
4131 Catawba Ridge
Gainesville, GA 30506
USA
aferris@emory.edu

ISSN 1387-6570
ISBN 978-90-481-9147-5   e-ISBN 978-90-481-9148-2
DOI 10.1007/978-90-481-9148-2
Springer Dordrecht Heidelberg London New York

Library of Congress Control Number: 2010929141

Printed on acid-free paper

Springer is part of Springer Science+Business Media (www.springer.com)

For their wisdom and vision for social indicators
and the quality of life

Eleanor Bernert Sheldon
Alex C. Michalos
Joseph M. Sirgy
Kenneth C. Land

Acknowledgements

Dr. Margaret Herrman contributed the section on conflict resolution (pp. 47–50). Adrienne Ferriss spent many hours editing this volume. My special thanks to her. John Ferriss helped keep my computer civil. Mary Jane Ghent assembled the Index. Rosemary Wood Dodd offered helpful advice. My appreciation to each of these. Any remaining errors are my sad fault.

– Abbott L. Ferriss

Contents

Introduction

*As for happiness, it has hardly more than one useful quality,
namely to make unhappiness possible. In our happiness, we
should form very sweet bonds, full of confidence and
attachment, in order that the sundering of them may cause us
that priceless rending of the heart which is called unhappiness.*
    –Marcel Proust, Remembrance of Things Past, The Past
    Recaptured.

Sorrow is better than laughter: for by the sadness of the countenance the heart is made
better.

–Ecclesiastes, 7:3

A general definition of civilization: a civilized society is exhibiting the five qualities of
Truth, Beauty, Adventure, Art, Peace.

–Alfred North Whitehead

The Social Environment

Following Bertrand Russell, this study proposes that a better quality of life (QOL),
a good life, will result from a better society, a good society. To improve the QOL,
the social and physical environments should be improved. The process will involve
some changes in the social structure and social psychology, cultural patterns, and
organization in some, but not all, communities. Interventions will be proposed to
bring about improvements. This is the purpose of this study.

The study identifies aspects of the social system that, when modified, will support
10 keys of the QOL. The ten domains of the QOL, in their way, affect individual,
family, community, and nation of the social system. Although individual-personal
considerations are discussed, I propose chiefly alterations in socioeconomic conditions that will improve the QOL.

The Community Indicators Consortium has shown that citizens working together
can change conditions for the better. In some instances, such as cigarette smoking,
governmental fiat has brought about change. Committees concerned with specific
local problems have effectively improved conditions. Whatever be the force for
change, it can be done by citizens working together. Knowing what to change is
the key.

The social, political, and economic organization of the society matter in creating an environment for a better QOL. A recent study of European nations supports the theory that "social settings turn out to be an influential domain for individual well-being." Life satisfaction is negatively affected in a social system that lacks trust in the political and welfare systems of the country. "Political and institutional settings are considered to be contextual frameworks which limit and structure the options and opportunities to take advantage of life chances" (Bohnke, 2008). This book explores the effects of the social environment on the QOL. It is a search for the social conditions making for the *good life*.

Veenhoven (2009) has marshaled happiness data for 92 nations along with length of life, happy life years, and enjoyment of life. He finds a strong correlation between these QOL measures and societal characteristics. The latter are government effectiveness, quality of regulations, control of corruption, and voice and accountability. He shows that people live better in nations that "flourish" best. Other societal measures also show strong association with QOL measures; these are biological capacity, economic competitiveness, military power, and integration into the world system. Political stability, ethnic fragmentation, and civil war, also, are included, the latter two being negatively associated with happy life years. Thus, within the limits of available data, Veenhoven's analysis gives ample support for the thesis of this book.

European scholars have theorized concerning the good life by identifying four components. These are *socioeconomic security, social inclusion, social cohesion*, and *social empowerment*. These components are values promoting the good life. A study using Israeli data found *socioeconomic security* positively associated with social inclusion but *socioeconomic security* was independent of social cohesion (Monnickendam & Berman, 2008). One would not expect this finding to be universal, since social systems have different organizational structures.

The economic system in modern industrial societies dominates as the basis of the good life. The production of wealth promotes the good life (Moss, 1979). Hence, the gross domestic product per capita has become the criterion of better living, despite its shortcomings. Only the small kingdom of Bhutan has set happiness as the criteria for determining change/progress. Identifying the social–organizational characteristics of a good society will move us closer to understanding and controlling influences upon the QOL.

Domains of the QOL

Domains of the QOL serve as a framework for propositions for change. Drawing upon the works of Abbey & Andres (1986), Mukherjee (1989), Ryff and Keyes (1995), Schwartz (1992, 1994), Keyes (1998), Ferriss (1990, 2000), Hagerty et al. (2000), Cummins (1996), Diener and Suh (1997), Diener (1995), (2005) and Ferriss (2001), I identified 10 domains that reflect a consensus of past scholarly work. The 10 domains are subject to modification in a specific society, depending upon the cultural norms that define the good life. Domains include survival of the species, social acceptance, mastery, affective autonomy, intellectual autonomy, egalitarian commitment, harmony, conservatism, hierarchy, and health. These 10 domains provide the framework of this study. In what follows, I shall define each of the 10 domains, show some redundancy among them, and state propositions that will point to a better QOL.

While the 10 domains were based upon the categories identified by numerous scholars of the QOL, they correspond in the main with categories developed by the Organisation for Economic Co-operation and Development (OECD) in the 1990s. OECD has promoted the development of national social reports and provided an outline of topics, which is essentially the same as the categories proposed as a comprehensive taxonomy of social quality. The OECD categories of social quality are listed below. The corresponding domains used herein are in parentheses.

Health – length of life, healthfulness of life (Survival, Health)

Education – use of educational facilities, learning (Intellectual Autonomy)

Employment – availability of employment, quality of working life (Mastery, Hierarchy)

Command over goods and services – income, wealth (Hierarchy)

Physical environment – housing conditions, access to services, environmental nuisances (Harmony)

Personal safety – exposure to risk, perceived threat (Conservatism)

Social environment – social attachment (Social Acceptance, Affective Autonomy)

Time and leisure – use of time (Egalitarian Commitment, Health)

The OECD categories were extracted from Berman and Philips (2000).

It is informative to also compare the QOL domains used herein with those of the widely used Australian Unity Well-Being Index (Cummins, Eckersley, Pallant, van Vugt, & Misajon, 2003). It employs a Personal Index of seven areas and a National Index of three, for a total of ten domains. The Personal Index includes Standard of Living, Health, Achievement, Relationships, Safety, Community, and Future Security. The National Index consists of Economic, State of the Environment, and Social Conditions. While the nomenclature differs, except for Health, the phenomena identified are the same as the domains herein used, as are the OECD categories.

Positive and Negative

Each domain presents both positive and negative features. For example, Survival of the Species is deterred by suicide, wars, disasters, and the like, while it is abetted by extending the length of life and a fertility rate higher than replacement. This text explores how negative features may be avoided or removed and how positive features may be enhanced.

Subjective, Objective

The QOL is indexed by both subjective and objective measures. Scholars gather responses to questionnaires that ask the respondent's satisfaction with life, job, family, leisure time, and other aspects of living. These measures reflect subjective well-being (SWB) and its correlates. Eid and Diener (2004) have examined the effect of mood on the questionnaire responses and concluded it minimally important. Happiness is also studied as a domain of SWB. These are subjective assessments of the QOL (Bramston, Pretty & Chipuer, 2002).

Objective measures of the QOL include health, income, conditions of housing and neighborhood, and other such characteristics as reported by the respondent and as reflected in averages of geographic units (city, county, enumeration district, etc.).

Subjective and objective measures do not always reveal the same level of QOL. Cummins (2000) has pointed out that the two must be considered separately and that objective measures do not reflect the happiness that SWB mirrors. In Taiwan, a 23 area study showed that only on Education and Environmental Quality were subjective and objective measures significantly associated. Other measures (medical service, domestic finances, work, leisure, public safety) were not significantly associated with subjective measures. However, the number of areas in the study, 23, is small and the result could be questioned because of sample size (Liao, 2009). In addition, the items included in the objective index may not reflect the conditions that generate the SWB response. The fact remains that some people's perception of their QOL may differ from others, even given the same physical surroundings. "Needs" and "wants" vary, sometimes being consistent and sometimes not.

QOL

Hajiran (2006), from an economic point of view, has proposed a definition of QOL. He sets forth the concept of a Net Domestic Product of Happiness. QOL is defined, in his words, "as the product of the interaction between an individual's personality and the continuous episodes of life events. The life events occur within a multidimensional set of domains, namely, liberty, knowledge, economics, health, safety, social relationships, spirituality, environment, and recreation" (p. 33). His nine domains are equivalent to the ten domains listed above, merely a difference in nomenclature (q.v. Ferriss, 2000). Being an economist, he proposes the use of the Law of Diminishing Marginal Utility (LDMU), which accounts as a utility the satisfaction or dissatisfaction (disutility) derived from life events. Needs are satisfied or not. He quotes Maslow's need hierarchy theory, as follows, "hierarchal pyramid of needs includes basic needs (food, shelter, safety), social needs (affection, belonging, acceptance), and ego needs (recognition, autonomy, achievement, self-actualization). Maslow's ego needs are the highest order of needs and are very similar to Aristotle's theory of happiness that emphasizes self-actualization and seeking happiness from within oneself, rather than extracting happiness from external and often transitory elements such as wealth" (pp. 37–38). He proposes to call the QOL measure the "Net Domestic Product of Happiness." He uses "net" because the positive values are to be diminished by the negative values. He proposes a summation of the nine domains, each measured objectively, using a common metric. Presumably, the nine domains have equal weight, but this is unclear. His ultimate goal, however, is "defining, evaluating, measuring, and enhancing QOL" by the social system.

One often hears QOL discussed in terms of happiness. What makes us happy? QOL involves more than happiness or sadness. But the "pursuit of happiness" has become a leading concept in QOL research.

Happiness

What is happiness? Ask, and you will get different answers. ". . .good health and bad memory," said Albert Schweitzer. "Happiness belongs to the self-sufficient," wrote Aristotle.

According to the psychoanalyst Carl Jung, "Even a happy life cannot be without a measure of darkness, and the word 'happy' would lose its meaning if it were not balanced by sadness." Melancholy is promoted as a counteractive to happiness in a recent book by Eric G. Wilson (2008). He believes that we become human through experience of joy and sorrow.

Claude Monet, the artist, found happiness arising from nature, which inspired his paintings. Love of work, also, is the basis for happiness according to others, including Francoise de Motteville and W. Beran Wolfe. But others are less down to earth. Sophocles puts his finger on wisdom, while Susan B. Anthony prefers independence as the basis for happiness.

"It's not money," said Franklin D. Roosevelt, but "the thrill of creative effort." ". . . (T)o love and be loved" generates happiness for the French writer George Sand. Something similar, compassion, is the basis of happiness for the Dalai Lama: ". . .our happiness arises in the context of our relationships with others," he adds. Similarly, James M. Barrie finds happiness in "bringing sunshine into the lives of others." Gandhi, the Indian leader and mystic, would find happiness in harmony "in what you think, what you say, and what you do."

Defining happiness has no end. The Harvard University psychologist Daniel Gilbert sees happiness as three aspects: emotional, moral, and judgmental (Gilbert, 2006). Brain neuroscientists have located the pleasures of happiness in the left prefrontal cortex of the brain. Sensations of sadness and unhappiness, of which Jung speaks, are located in the right prefrontal cortex. It is good to know that happiness and unhappiness are located in the brain, but how do they get there? Undoubtedly, our external behaviors, reactions, and relationships form the basis of the satisfactions, dissatisfactions, pleasures, and disappointments that generate happiness or sorrow.

These eclectic definitions of happiness illustrate the variety of understandings of the QOL. As a major aspect of the SWB, happiness will be discussed later as we dissect the QOL in its many dimensions (see Chapter 4).

Chapter 1
Survival of the Species

"What are we fighting for?"
Then, then we'll end that stupid crime,
When we, the Workers, all demand:
That devil's madness – war.

–Robert William Service, Michael

The survival of the fittest which I have here sought to express in mechanical terms is that which Mr. Darwin has called "natural selection, or the preservation of favored races in the struggle for life."

Herbert Spencer, Principles of Biology (1864–1867), Indirect Equilibration

There has never been a war yet which, if the facts had been put calmly before the ordinary folk, could not have been prevented. The common man is the greatest protection against war.

Ernest Bevin, Speech, House of Commons, November 1945

The Survival of the Species. The Survival of the Species requires fertility levels adequate to assure continuation of the species. Environmental contaminants, wars, intergroup conflict such as religious pogroms, and other impediments that deplete population must be reduced or eliminated.

Proposition 1. The QOL may be enhanced by reducing negative survival features, such as suicide, homicides, wars, and terrorist intrusions, and by achieving a fertility rate greater than replacement, usually considered to be 2.1 lifetime births per woman.

Scholars usually do not identify survival of the species as a domain of the QOL. However, Mukherjee (1989) identified this element in his review of the works of major social scientists. Several domain sets imply it in lists of life conditions. In commenting on Schwartz' (1992, 1994) overview of universal values, Diener (1995) reported, "These values represent the universal requirements of human existence: meeting needs, coordinated social interaction, and the survival and welfare needs of groups."

Mukherjee (1989), in an extensive survey of literature, identified values that define the "good life." He identified "cardinal valuations" of human kind in the works of W.I. Thomas, Robert S. Lind, L.L. Thurstone, A.H. Maslow, and others. Mukherjee's QOL index included four domains: "the survival of the species, security in the life span of humans, material prosperity for well-being, and mental progress to unfold the potentials of all individuals belonging to the species."

We in western civilization seldom consider the possibility that we or our progeny will no longer exist, yet in recent times there are population segments that have been reduced in size if not extinguished entirely. Examples are natural disasters, such as the 2004 tidal wave in the Indian Ocean northwest of Sumatra that killed nearly one-quarter million natives of four countries, and man-made pogroms, such as the 1933–1945 holocaust that extinguished an estimated six million. Large numbers have been devastated, if not eliminated completely. Below, some of the threats to survival are discussed, as well as a review of factors that, if followed, would help the human species survive.

Factors Leading to Extension

Individuals value survival of their immediate kin and the survival of the next level of kin, and the associates of their kin. Survival means the continuation of their heritage both biological and cultural. Charles Darwin described the natural selection process that operates in primitive societies to the end that the weak and infirm die early, leaving the "fitter" to survive and perpetuate their kind. This leads to a genetic inheritance with better survival probability. However, in civilized societies, the infirm and mentally, intellectually, and developmentally disabled individuals are not prevented from bearing children, leading to a diminished genetic pool (Zanner, 2002). One answer is to prevent the weak from reproducing and to encourage the well-endowed to have more offspring. However, in a democratic society, such eugenics policies are morally repugnant. Those apparently better endowed by standards of achievement in education, commerce, the arts, etc., have low birth rates.

The evolutionary process identified by Darwin and Wallace continues to this day, as human kind modifies and adapts to an ever-changing socio-cultural environment. Biologists have identified numerous genetic adaptations of modern man. According to McAuliffe (2008), (2009), ethnic groups are diverging rather than converging in traits. Biologists say many aspects of humankind are changing: "the brain, the digestive system, life span, immunity to pathogens, sperm production, and bones – in short, virtually every aspect of our functioning" (p. 51). In deciphering DNA, scientists have begun to identify the genetic basis of traits. Combined with cultural values, these changes challenge our idea of what constitutes the good life. Our ideas of the QOL likewise may be changing.

Fertility

Demographers view replacement fertility as essential for survival.

Their research on demographic change has uncovered the dynamics of the demographic transition. Population change transpires through the influence of industrialization, individualization, modernization, etc., and fertility changes from high, above replacement to low, below replacement. This demographic transition determines the rate of population growth or decline.

Many westernized countries now are below replacement. In a recent year, the total fertility rate for Europe was an average of 1.4 births per woman in her lifetime. Compare this with the 2.1 lifetime births per female required for replacement. For optimum QOL, we must consider the population size consistent with the carrying capacity (economic, biological, social) of the area (nation). Public policies in rapidly growing nations have effectively altered fertility through limiting births to reduce population growth, as in China's one-child per couple policy. Aware of a dwindling population, other countries turn to stimulating fertility, as in Sweden, through policies that enable working women to receive child benefits, provisions to leave paid work temporarily to care for the newborn, restrictions on abortion, artificial insemination, in vitro fertilization, surrogate motherhood, and other such innovative technologies (Nam, 1994). In short, survival of the species with optimum QOL may be assured by public policies that affect fertility and population growth when it is consonant with the carrying capacity of the economy.

Fertility of women is inversely related to women's education (Nam, 1994, p. 192). Women's education and higher socioeconomic status (SES) have been associated with lower fertility. Recently, higher SES families have increased their fertility slightly, leading to better quality of offspring. "We assume that SES is associated with genetic quality, but we know also the differential effects on fertility of age, period, cohort, religion, region, and other factors" (Matras, 1977, p. 192). Thus, improving the status and QOL of females will result in lower fertility and slower population growth.

Fertility has declined in many newly industrialized countries. For example, Singapore has a below replacement rate of 1.2 births per woman. European countries have fertility rates below replacement. South Korea has the lowest birth rate with 1.1 per woman. The Korean government has instituted measures to reverse the decline in the birth rate, including improved maternity leave, subsidies for childcare, and "baby bonuses." A family and gender expert, however, has recommended more long-range strategies, such as improving the economic conditions of young people of child-bearing ages, supporting egalitarian gender roles, and reducing the cost of children's education. These policies are designed to increase fertility while improving the QOL.

Higher child mortality appears to encourage higher fertility. Infant mortality in Africa is 86 per 1,000 live births, while its total fertility rate stands at 5.2. By contrast, infant mortality in Europe is 8 per 1,000 live births, while its total fertility rate is below replacement, 1.4. The consequence of these and many other economic, social, and political factors results in a low-fertility rate in developed countries. Developed countries have a total fertility rate of 1.6; this contrasts with a rate of 3.1 in less-developed countries. By 2050, Europe and North America will decline as a proportion of the world population from 17 to 11%, while Africa and Asia will increase from 74% in the year 2000 to 80% of the world population in 2050 (Haub, 2002; O'Neil & Balk, 2001).

High fertility in less-developed countries presents a major problem in population control. Excessive population growth that is not accompanied by economic growth leads to lower QOL. On the other hand, low fertility and low population growth is a problem in European countries. There, women are in the labor force. Children's education and socialization has become a state function. Peer influence upon children becomes dominant compared with family influence, leading to increased delinquency, use of drugs and related behaviors. Fertility, consequently, has ramifications beyond mere population growth.

Public policies may intervene. Currently, low fertility countries are unlikely to stimulate fertility, as was done by Germany, prior to and during World War II, and by Sweden, as population policy in the 1930s. Experts view family survival as a familial concern rather than a matter for public policy (McNicoll, 2001). However, in the interest of survival, steps to improve fertility among families that can produce offspring and provide satisfactory QOL for them are needed. In the long run, zero population growth is the desirable policy.

Factors Leading to Exhaustion

Suicide

From several theories of suicide, let us first review those of Emile Durkheim (2002, recent edition) who reasoned that egoistic suicide results from a lack of the individual's integration in social groups. Durkheim believed that in people detached from society, the individual ego becomes predominant, supplanting the social ego, and the person thus separated from social controls commits suicide. The remedy for this, Durkheim stated, is to improve the group ties – religious, familial, economic – such that the individual is influenced by the norms of these constructive groups.

Altruistic suicide results from the individual's being so extensively integrated into the group norms that the person gives his life for the benefit of the group. This is observed in war when a soldier gives his life to prevent danger to his fellow soldiers. Terrorist acts of suicide by religious fundamentalists also may be interpreted to result from such intense integration into the norms of a group (norms that reward suicide) that the person gives his life to bring benefit to the religious group and himself through the promise of eternal after-life bliss. The norms of the social group are critical in altruistic suicide.

Fatalistic suicide results from social ties that lead to despondency. Anomic suicide arises from unspecific norms and weak social support. The remedy for this, Durkheim reasoned, is, as above, to improve the group ties – religious, familial, economic – such that the individual is influenced by the norms of constructive groups. Helliwell (2007) examined suicide and social capital in 50 countries to see if Durkheim's early study of suicide conclusions by country would hold up in 1990. It did, despite the increase in suicide rates in most countries, especially in Russia and Finland. Helliwell also found SWB and social capital, belief in God, and volunteerism tend to increase life satisfaction and a reduction in suicide rates. In short, a satisfactory QOL accompanied by close group association will decrease suicide (Bronisch, 2001).

Other theories of suicide focus upon the psychological state of the person. S. Freud assumed that aggression against the ego resulted in devaluation of self, and hence, suicide. A.T. Beck's theories focus upon depression as the basis for suicide, while H. Henseler found that narcissistic persons, hurt by others, react irrationally, leading to aggressive outbursts against others or self, sometimes resulting in suicide.

To reduce the frequency of suicide, we must consider the type of suicide. In general, the instrument for reducing suicide is to enhance the social bond of individuals to the family and other groups that provide a reason for living, and to reduce the attachment of the individual to groups that advocate altruistic suicide. These theories are further elaborated by Joseph (2003, pp. 79–83).

Disease

People of primitive cultures, especially those in Africa, suffer the ravages of diseases that threaten survival (Hijab, 2007). Malaria, for example, kills some two million children annually in Africa. Families that normally would limit births to two or three, instead, because of the threat of malaria, have six or seven to ensure survival of the family. Thus, paradoxically, malarial mortality stimulates fertility. Quinine is the traditional remedy that checks fever and chills of malaria. Now, medicines based upon artemisinin, an extract of a Chinese herb, effectively treat the disease at a cost of about US $1. However, when a child becomes ill, poor families cannot afford treatment. A preventive step includes the mosquito net, which costs approximately $10, again prohibitive to poor families. Jeffrey D. Sachs, author of *The End of Poverty*, estimates that the disease throughout Africa could be controlled at a cost of $4.50 per person, which comes to three billion dollars annually. Information on active programs is available on the Internet at www.malarianomore.com and www.nothingbutnets.net.

Jay Keasling, a chemical engineer at the University of California at Berkeley, has developed synthetic artemisinin. His work is supported by a 43 million dollar grant from the Bill and Melinda Gates Grant Foundation. As an engineer, biologist, and chemist, Keasling has engaged genetic engineering to initiate the new field of synthetic biology, which employs yeast and other substances to form a factory that reduces the cost of producing artemisinin. It holds promise of an economical treatment of malaria. Production by 2010 is expected (Zimmer, Dunn, & Kahn, 2006).

Another scourge in Africa and Asia has been Guinea worm disease, caused by drinking water contaminated by the worm. In 1986, three experts estimated 3.5 million cases in 20 countries. In that year, the Carter Center began a program to eradicate the disease. Now, over 20 years later, experts say the disease is 99.7% eradicated. Two funds – the Bill and Melinda Gates Foundation and the United Kingdom Department for International Development – have donated $55 million to complete the eradication of the Guinea worm.

These two examples illustrate the effect of concerted effort supported by adequate funds. The world, however, is beset by many other diseases that detract from the QOL. Among them is HIV/AIDS. Epidemic levels of the disease have been reached in southern Asia and sub-Saharan Africa. India and China show lower rates, but the number infected in India alone is more than four million. Once a plague, smallpox has since been almost entirely eliminated. Public health programs, better personal sanitation, improved food supply, and other factors have reduced mortality from many infectious diseases (Harris, 2007).

Disasters

In geologic meaures, mass extinction of the earth's life has occurred at least 20 times. There have been at least five major catastrophic extinctions and at least 14 other events that affected loss of at least 20% of the Earth's species. Natural disasters happen, and future devastations are possible.

Man-made and natural disasters kill many people. During the 7-year-period ending in 2006, man-made accidents killed an average of more than 3,435 annually worldwide, excluding automobile accidents (which are reported only for the US). These were accidents involving aircraft, ships, trains, fires, explosions, or stampedes.

Natural disasters were more violent, an average of 62,706 persons dying annually because of tornadoes, hurricanes, typhoons, blizzards, floods, tsunamis, summer heat (in Europe), and earthquakes during the above-mentioned 7 years. The total is more than 462,300. (These data may not be inclusive, for they are from newspaper accounts.)

Storms, cyclones, tornadoes, and hurricanes devastate areas from time to time. In spring of 2008, southern Myanmar (formerly Burma), they took an estimated 128,000 lives. Other recent disasters:

Typhoon, Iris, Vietnam, 1964, 7,000 lives
Typhoon, Thelma, Philippines, 1991, 5,956 lives
Typhoon, Linda, Vietnam, 2007, 3,682 lives
Cyclone, Myanmar, 1926, 2,700 lives
Cyclone, Indonesia, 1973, 1,650 lives
Tropical Storm, Philippines, 2004, 1,619 lives

In addition to these estimates of lives lost, we must consider the living, whose QOL was diminished by loss of homes, employment, food, and living conditions. Often, illness follows storms, owing to unsanitary conditions and lack of clean drinking water. Following such natural disasters, the United Nations and various countries contribute aid, such as tents, rice, cooking utensils, and other necessities. These efforts often are coordinated by the United Nations agencies. Natural disasters deplete the QOL (Gill, 2007).

Government meteorology services may issue warning of the approaching storm. This may help when it is possible for people to move away from the expected impact. Governments, however, do not always warn their people soon enough. People cannot always escape to safe haven. Living in an area free of danger provides the safest insurance. Otherwise, early warning and the provision of transportation are the most that can be done to cushion the impact of natural disasters. Clean up and assistance with rebuilding may help restore the QOL to some degree (Kaplan, 2008).

War

Beyond these natural disasters, humankind has suffered "the devil's madness", war. As the technology of killing has become more efficient, war has become more and more damaging to human existence. War is the most significant institution affecting survival. Large segments of a generation, usually young men, are killed. This alters the gene pool in unfathomable ways. The effect on the sequence of generations continues for decades. The effect of the War Between the States continued into the twentieth century, because of the size of the cohort that was not born because of the conflict. War is the most devastating, preventable impact upon the QOL. During the twentieth century, countries formally declared war on others on 250 occasions. Estimates of deaths exceed 100 million. Political repression, communal violence, and genocide took millions more (Nordstrom, 2001).

Efforts to reduce conflict between nations and within nations have become one of the primary functions of the United Nations. During 2007, the UN maintained 18 peacekeeping missions worldwide. During the 1980s and 1990s in Sudan, the southerners, chiefly Christians, took up arms against government domination. The chiefly Arab–Muslim conflict caused an estimated two million deaths. Amnesty International declared that the basis of the conflict was "ethnic cleansing." During 2003–2006, rebellion arose in the Darfur region of western Sudan. An estimated 200,000 were killed, some two million fled to refugee camps (Kashner, 2007), and we are still counting.

During the twentieth century and the first 7 years of the 21st, US casualties resulting from principal wars exceeded 2,065,736. This includes non-mortal wounded as well as deaths. Total US personnel involved in these conflicts exceeded 36 million (Kashner, 2007). War impacts the QOL in countless ways – economically, genetically, socially, psychologically, and intellectually.

Genocide

Outright genocide by one political or cultural faction against another, or the imposing of famine, resulted in at least 17 million deaths during the twentieth century. The number includes the 1915 extermination of Armenians by Turks (more than a million), a famine in the Ukraine during the 1930s (six or seven million), the

1933–1945 holocaust of the Nazi party against the Jews (an estimated six million), the 1975–1979 extermination in Cambodia under Pol Pot of the Khmer rouge (estimated 1.5–2.0 million), the 1988 campaign of the Iraqi government against the Kurds (estimated up to 200,000), the 1992–1995 killing of Bosnian Muslims by Serbs after the breakup of Yugoslavia (200,000), the 1994 massacre of Tutsis by Hutus in Rwanda (800,000), and the 2003 to the present attacks of the Sudan government and rebel groups against blacks and non-Arab southern tribes in the Darfur region (800,000 and counting). These estimates do not include the purges instigated by Joseph Stalin in Russia that took an estimated 20 million lives. Other estimates of genocide victims in the Soviet Union from 1917–1987 are 40–60 million. The Chinese Cultural Revolution is said to have cost several million lives. Red China under Mao before 1949 caused 40–60 million casualties (Kashner, 2007, p. 125; Naimark, 2001). Since World War II, many other nations have suffered genocide: Poland, 1.4 million, Czechoslovakia, 240,000, Ethiopia, 4 million, Albania, 10,000, and communist Germany, some 9,000 (Nordstrom, 2001).

More than 130 nations have agreed to the Convention on the Prevention and Punishment of the Crime of Genocide, set up in 1951. Although termed "crimes against humanity," the Nazi trials at Nuremberg were for crimes based on religious or racial grounds. The UN Security Council set up tribunals to try perpetrators of genocide and other crimes in the former Yugoslavia and Rwanda. In 2002, the International Criminal Court began trials of genocide crimes. Legal machinery, thus, is in place to enforce universal opposition to genocide. The deliberate destruction of a group based upon religious, ethnic, or racial factors demeans humanity and depletes life and the QOL.

Religious Conflict

An aspect of genocide, conflict between religious organizations has led to untold misery and death. Currently, at least a dozen conflicts disturb the peace of the world. Jews are contending with Muslims in Israel–Palestine, Muslims oppose Hindus in Kashmir. In the Sudan, Muslims are fighting Christians and animists; they are against Christians, also, in Nigeria. In Indonesia, Muslims are against the Timorese Christians; in the Caucasus, Chechen Muslims are against Orthodox Russians, and Muslim Azerbaijanis oppose Catholic and Orthodox Armenians. In Sri Lanka, Sinhalese Buddhists oppose Tamil Hindus, and in the Balkans, Orthodox Serbians are poised against Catholic Croatians and Bosnian and Albanian Muslims. In Northern Ireland, the struggle has somewhat abated between the Protestants and Catholics (Harris, 2004), thanks to the efforts of George Mitchell. Theological differences haunt the world, despite an ethic of peace and brotherhood in most theological doctrines. Religious leaders of contending doctrines should sit down together to work out differences and reach out to peace.

Tribal Extinction

Anthropologists have canvassed causes of tribal extinction and have identified the following as chief causes: lack of nutrients, disease, genetic abnormalities, unusual weather, being out-competed for natural resources, changes in climate (Texler, 2006). Jared Diamond (2005), an environmental biologist, has identified five factors causing extinction of societies: climate change, human environmental impact, hostile neighbors, decreased support from friendly neighbors, failure of a society to respond adequately to environmental problems. Diamond's book documents historical occasions of society's collapse.

Language experts have documented the extinction or loss of language by tribes, but a more dominant language may be adopted by a tribe without losing its identity. It is not a reliable means of counting extinct tribes.

Family Violence

Aggression among family members may become a divisive factor in family relations and may lead to their breakup, thereby destroying the potential for family succession. Frustration over sometimes trivial family concerns, budgets, work schedules, extra-social activities, and the like may lead to aggression of one family member against another. Frustration also may arise from relationships at work, entirely outside the family circle, and lead to displaced aggression against family members. Psychologists have also identified other types of aggression: relational aggression, instrumental or proactive aggression, passive aggression, and affective aggression.

The Center for Disease Control and Prevention released a study in May 2008, showing that domestic violence was a factor in 52% of female homicides and 9% of male homicides. Unhappy family relationships, also, is a motive for leaving home and becoming homeless. Neighbors' intervention in domestic violence poses both a benefit and a risk. Hearing loud voices next door may lead a neighbor to intervene, risking violence against the neighbor. The National Network to End Domestic Violence recommends that neighbors inform victims of hotlines and shelters to which victims may retire. This should be done when the abuser is not present. The victim should keep a bag packed with toilet, personal items, a checkbook, and other essentials, prepared to move to a shelter. The victim should know to signal a neighbor or to phone police when their presence is appropriate. In some cities, such as San Francisco, there is a Family Violence Prevention Fund to aid victims.

Psychologists do not advise suppressing frustration or anger. Suppression leads to higher blood pressure and risks of heart problems. Expression is preferred, but the mode of expression is important. It is best for the person aroused "to express his or her feelings clearly but without hostility" and to discuss the situation calmly to seek a mutually satisfactory solution to the source of frustration and aggression

(Green, 1999). Of course, in the heat of anger, this may not occur to the parties. An intermediary might initiate the steps of conflict resolution (see Chapter 5 on conflict resolution.)

Conclusion: Factors Promoting Survival

For conflict between nations, international tribunals are in place to bring perpetuators to justice, the United Nations being the primary instrument. The leaders of political or religious bodies have responsibilities to reduce friction and bring about peace. Their efforts are essential if the QOL is to be improved.

On a more intimate level, conflict resolution has proven itself beneficial in bringing contending parties into a solution of problems. Applying it to family violence will reduce this threat to survival. This requires patience, time, and acceptance of ethical principals of justice, equality, and consideration of others.

Adjusting to climate change through international understandings that reduce environmental contaminants would go far toward reducing change and insuring a better base for improved QOL.

War, genocide, conflict between theological adherents, and other such sources of international hostility deplete the resources for a better QOL. With world population growing toward more than nine billion, such sources of strife will likely increase. Diplomacy, civility, and unceasing vigilance of all nations are needed to reduce strife and maintain peace in the larger population of the future.

We must anticipate and adapt to natural disasters, minimizing their impact through advanced warning and moving the people from harms way. Man-made disasters arise chiefly from the machine, which brings us many benefits as well. We know that diseases with effort may be overcome through medical and public health efforts. We also know that time, effort, and financial resources are required. International understandings and concerted efforts are needed.

As Thomas Paine (1737–1809) expressed it: "I believe that religious duties consist in doing justice, loving mercy, and endeavoring to make our fellow-creatures happy." –*The Age of Reason,* Part I.

Chapter 2
Social Acceptance

Self-reverence, self-knowledge, self-control,
These three alone lead life to sovereign power.
–Alfred, Lord Tennyson, Oerone (1833), line 142

Dissatisfaction with the world in which we live and determination to realize one that shall be better, are the prevailing characteristics of the modern spirit.
–Goldsworthy Lowes Dickinson, The Greek View of Life, Ch. 5

Great God, I ask thee for no meaner pelf
Than that I may not disappoint myself,
That in my action I may soar as high
As I can now discern with this clear eye.
–Henry David Thoreau, A Prayer (1842), Stanza 1

Social Acceptance: Positive Self-Concept. Emotional well-being involves positive feelings about past experience. Low self-acceptance involves dissatisfaction with self, disappointment with past attainments. Participation in group activities, attending religious gatherings, or engaging in constructive leisure activities, sports, etc., support the development of world view and enhances the ego.

Proposition 2. The QOL may be enhanced by minimizing dissatisfaction with the self and disappointment over past actions and augmenting emotional well-being through positive experiences, participation in ego-enhancing group activities, developing a world view, and acquiring a purpose in life through education and spiritual conditioning.

Mental Health

Corey Keyes (1998) introduced the concept of "flourishing" as an indicator of mental health. "Flourishing is a combination of two very ancient traditions of views of happiness. Aristotle thought it was just positive functioning; Epicurus thought it was just feeling good. It turns out that to flourish is to feel good and function well in life," Keyes said. He outlined 13 characteristics of flourishing, signs of positive mental health: (1) positive emotions; (2) avowed satisfaction with life; (3) making a contribution to society; (4) social integration; (5) social growth and potential;

(6) acceptance of others; (7) social interest and coherence; (8) self-acceptance; (9) environmental mastery (control); (10) positive relations with others; (11) personal growth; (12) autonomy; (13) having a purpose in life. These and other characteristics of flourishing are also discussed in Chapters 3, Mastery, and 4, Affective Autonomy.

The Keyes model was tested by Joshanloo and Nosratabadi (2009) with a sample of 227 Iranian university students. They reported that four personality traits successfully distinguished three mental-health dimensions (flourishing, moderately healthy, and languishing). Neuroticism, extraversion, and conscientiousness discriminated between the flourishing and languishing groups. Persons of moderate mental health scored higher on agreeableness. Openness, as a personality trait, failed to distinguish the mental-health dimensions. Thus, these personality traits support some of the 13 dimensions that Keyes identified for positive mental health. These traits, like a good meal, generate satisfaction with life and a better QOL.

Spiritual Experiences

Self-acceptance and enhancement of the self involve spiritual experiences. These include social service activities, participation in religious activities, worship, and service to others. Spiritual qualities, like compassion for others, empathy, altruism, and kindness make for the *good life*. Such spiritual capital contributes to better health, lower blood pressure, lower rates of lung and stomach cancer, and the like. Persons ranking high on spiritual capital tend to have stronger immune systems. These are among the health benefits of religious participation and spiritual capital. Religious organizations influence behavior through enforcing rules against unhealthy habits, such as cigarette smoking, use of alcohol, caffeine, etc. These restrictions, like mother always said, make for healthier living (Wortham & Wortham, 2007).

A study of 459 college students (Zullig, Ward, & Horn, 2006) found students high in spirituality also high in self-perceived health, with higher life satisfaction. The authors think religiosity influences self-perceived health and the conditions making for better physical health, such as freedom from infections, pain, colds, etc. The three are intertwined – spirituality, life satisfaction, and perceived health. The authors find that good health promotes life satisfaction.

In a sample of young Estonian university students, a question on the meaningfulness of life yielded significant correlations on psychological well-being and moderate correlations with physical health and social relationships. The authors (Teichmann, Murdvee, & Saks, 2006) acknowledge the possible influence on the young sample of the socioeconomic shift from socialist economic relations to a free market economy. The tendency, they say, is toward more materialistic values. Nevertheless, the meaningfulness of life question correlated highly ($r = 0.63$) with psychological well-being, an indicator of the QOL. Among the young people, the QOL index, as measured by the World Health Organization Index, also yielded a high correlation, $r = 0.64$, with meaningfulness of life. Thus, in a changing socioeconomic environment, the young are finding meaning in life with spirituality as its source.

Lower Mortality

Hummer, Rogers, Nam, and Elison (1999) conducted an extensive study that followed a representative US sample of 2,016 persons for 9 years. It established mortality rates. Religious persons live longer, even when the effects of age, sex, race, region, self-reported health, marital status and other social ties, cigarette smoking, being overweight, and consuming alcohol were held constant.

Trends

Grant (2008) developed a "Religiosity Index" that shows trends, 1952–2005, for the US. Historically, religiosity increased to about the mid-1960 s, declined to 1980, and after that, continued an irregular decline to 2003. In an unpublished study by Mazen Elfrakhani of the University of Texas, Austin, a trend in "no religion" in the US between 1972 and 2006 showed a distinct rise at about a 45° angle beginning in 1990. These distinctive religious trends do not follow the happiness trend for the country, which has been irregularly leveled (see Chapter 4, Affective Autonomy).

A study over 7 years, 1998–2004, found a positive relation between a Daily Spiritual Experience Scale (DSES) and psychological well-being. This was a period of rapid decline of the Religiosity Index, mentioned above. During this period, the study showed happiness and excitement with life fairly constant, while depression increased. DSES remained relatively constant, a mean of 3.90–4.01, from 1998 to 2004, the "theistic" component of DSES remaining constant while the "nontheistic" increased slightly (Ellison & Fan, 2008). The short span of time covered by this study shows some support for the change in religiosity and its relation to well-being. Despite the inconsistent dates of the trend, the fact remains that practice and belief in religion varies over time and currently is declining. While the factors responsible for the decline remain uncertain, scholars have suggested that the discoveries of science concerning the universe and the findings of historical studies of religious testaments may have weakened belief and faith.

Social System

Estonia represents an interesting aspect of spirituality. A former socialist system, it is currently adapting open-market values and finding itself in a state of cognitive dissonance (entertaining contrasting ideas), leading to psychological tension. In this milieu, personal beliefs are changing. People are pondering the meaning of life. Spirituality is highly associated with the QOL index in Estonia. However, only moderate association was found between spirituality and the several domains of

QOL (physical health, psychological well-being, independence, social relationships, and environment). Two samples showed QOL and spirituality correlated reasonably highly, $r = 0.64$ and 0.53. The study by Teichmann and others (2006) reflects the association between QOL and spirituality in a changing socioeconomic environment. People look for lasting values and assurances, as they also look for the security of home and fireside.

We conclude that the self-concept and self-acceptance is enhanced through participation in activities of a spiritual nature, acquiring spiritual capital.

Family

Child Socialization

In the family, socialization of the child should build self-confidence and other supporting personality characteristics. The disruption of family life affects the present and several subsequent generations, for family social traits are passed on to succeeding generations. Creating harmonious relationships within the family, then, is a positive step toward self-acceptance.

Family structure makes a difference. Studies have shown that single-parent families, as opposed to husband–wife ones, are more likely to produce offspring that grow up to enter disruptive marital relationships, divorce, etc. For example, a New Zealand study tracing family QOL characteristics, 1981–2001, found that the country's efforts to improve conditions had little impact upon one-parent families (Cottrell, Weldon, & Mulligan, 2008). In addition, children who were abused by family members were more likely to become adults who abuse their offspring. Families should strive to rear children so as to secure the child's self-esteem.

Parents should support children, encouraging them to "constructively express their feelings, taking an interest in children's activities, showing respect for their children's point of view, and teaching their children how to exercise self-control and handle responsibility" (Lauer & Lauer, 2006, p. 359). To break the destructive habits which pass from generation to generation in family life, then, requires reorienting parents from their inherited patterns of discipline and self-control to more harmonious relationships within their families. This can be accomplished through parental education, beginning with the arrival of the first child. Witness the revolution, actually, in childcare generated by Dr. Spock's instructive volume which taught many post-World War II generations. Parent education is needed to create harmonious families. Adult education should take place through community organizations and religious groups.

Offspring Defects

Families may face unanticipated, trying problems. A child may be born with congenital defects, such as a missing ventricle of the heart, an improperly connected colon, or some disorder discovered developmentally, such as autism, type one diabetes, or a psychogenic disorder. Some of these problems may be corrected surgically, while others may require extended medical attention with associated costs. The husband, wife, and other sibling(s) face continuing problems of adjustment. In some cases, the family may be unable to cope and is dissolved by divorce with consequent reduction in the QOL. In others, family members may join forces and work toward a resolution of the child's problem. Supporting one another and suffering hardship together may lead to greater integrity of the family. In one such example, a child's cardiovascular problem was resolved after three operations. The husband reported that the episode brought him and his wife closer, resulting in improved QOL, that he rated 9.5 on a 10-point scale.

Homosexuality

Some families must cope with the social biases related to homosexuality in their offspring. While the cause of homosexuality remains under study, genetic or hormonal factors may have created brain differences while the fetus is in the womb. In *Proceedings* of *the National Academy of Science*, studies have identified structural brain similarities between homosexual men and heterosexual women. They report similarity in the brain area involving language. The neurobiologist Simon LeVay found that the hypothalamus in gay men is smaller than that of straight men. Gay men have symmetrical brains, similar to those of straight women. These distinguishing brain differences, then, provide immutable evidence of the condition. Families need to adjust by accepting the condition. Accepting the unalterable would contribute to the gay person's QOL and improve social inclusion of the community.

Likewise, the community needs to accept the condition. Community acceptance has greatly improved in recent years, leading to a social environment more supportive of the gay personality. But much remains to be done. Gay couples desire legal and social conditions equal to those of regularly married couples, but society thus far has been reluctant to grant them. The legality of marriage of gay couples in California recently has been revoked. This area of social acceptance remains for the future. Scientists' findings provide the rationale for accepting the gay/lesbian condition. Such rational acceptance would lead to improved QOL of the families involved and the gay persons, welcoming them home like the prodigal son.

Teen Pregnancy

Adolescence may be a trying period in the life of females. Their need for self-acceptance and recognition has caused an increase in pregnancy among 15-year-old girls in Gloucester, MA, according to news reports. Authorities say the girls' desire to be pregnant arises from low self-esteem and lack of hope. They believe that sex education and teaching methods to prevent pregnancy do not address the problem of low self-esteem. The girls need guidance from experienced hands to help them understand that staying in school and contributing to the community are more important than expressing their sexuality through out-of-wedlock pregnancy. A support network for them is important. This is another example of how the self-concept affects the QOL.

Margaret Talbot (2008) analyzed the teen-pregnancy condition in terms of conservative/liberal politics and egalitarian/liberal religion. Politically conservative families prefer that their pregnant out-of-wedlock daughter bring the fetus to full term rather than abort. Getting married and taking responsibility for the child is the ideal. Even so, social conservatives promote abstinence-only education and favor waiting until marriage for sex. Most evangelical teenagers believe in abstaining from sex before marriage. Despite this, evangelical teens are more likely than mainline Protestants, Mormons, and Jews to be sexually active and are less likely to employ contraception. Adolescent teens in close-knit families that include both parents are more likely to delay intercourse out-of-wedlock. Politically, teen pregnancy rates are higher in conservative states than in more liberal environments. More likely, use of abortion may be the reason. Taking a pledge to refrain from sex until marriage has succeeded in delaying sex time-wise, but, nevertheless, more than half of those making such pledges have sex before marriage, according to Talbot (2008).

Turning now to possible solutions, it appears that abstinence-only education is unrealistic for teenagers. Preaching contraceptive use may be wiser. Close-knit families, well integrated, are more likely to protect the teenager. The political/religious environment has an impact, but the sexual well-being of the teen should be considered first. The aim should be to build emotionally resilient young families, stable and productive of a desirable QOL.

Friendship

The power of friendship, group membership, social support, and related social relationships have positive health consequences and lower mortality, according to a review of research by Benson (1996, pp. 180–181).

The self-concept evolves through interaction with others. It is a kind of circular process. One observes the reaction of others to one's behavior; from this, one acquires an idea of the kind of person one is. Then one attempts to meet the other's expectation. One develops a constructive self-concept by successful, positive relations with others.

Group Participation

Participation in groups creates opportunities for rewards and ego-enhancing activities, resulting in self-esteem and a positive self-concept. We may test the theory in various age-related situations (Baumeister & Tenge, 2003). Self-fulfillment results, in part, from success in achieving goals that one sets for one's self (Ferrara, 2001).

A recent Canadian study (Muhajarine, 2008) introduces the concept of neighborliness, showing that it has a positive effect upon QOL and self-related health. The sense of attachment to the local area and participation has a strong positive impact.

Living in a neighborhood with others of the same racial/ethnic identity affects the social support one enjoys and, for some ethnic groups, contributes to well-being. A study by Yuan (2008) of a sample of 2,482 Illinois respondents found that in same-race neighborhoods of Blacks but not Hispanics, social support improved. However, both Blacks and Hispanics enjoyed better emotional well-being in neighborhoods consisting largely of the same racial/ethnic group. Higher social support for Blacks in same-race neighborhoods appears to decrease depression and increase emotional well-being. However, this was not found for Hispanics in their chiefly Hispanic neighborhoods. A cultural factor appears to be operating. The authors did not include job or other discrimination in the study, but they reason that it may be a factor affecting Blacks, who enjoy non-discrimination relationships among their own kind. This was not the case with Hispanics. Scientist have yet to identify the exact mechanism, but they assume that within the same-race/ethnic neighborhood, discrimination is less likely, residents share common norms and values, and social isolation is lower with an improved sense of belonging. In three studies, Yuan identified the structural factors that influenced social support.

Across European countries, the frequency of interacting with others varies. The frequency of such interactions, however, is moderately associated with happiness. In two of Kafetsios'(2006) studies, frequency of social meetings was not associated with happiness and satisfaction. In England, characterized as an individualistic society, a higher level of social interaction was observed than in Greece, an evolving collectivist society. Spain and Portugal, on the other hand, showed higher frequencies of social interaction. The level of social interaction, therefore, affects the benefit of social support. The study also found that social support does not always generate positive results; it can be associated with anxiety and distress. Kafetstios also found age to be influential, with older people being happier than younger ones. Thus, we cannot assume that social support in all circumstances will generate greater satisfaction and happiness; it depends upon cultural factors, social-organizational influences, frequency of participation, and age of participants. The poet John Keats (1795–1821) expressed it thus

> Wherein lies happiness? In that which becks
> Our ready minds to fellowship divine,
> A fellowship with essence; till we shine,
> Full achemiz'd, and free of space. Behold
> The clear religion of heaven!

Group Structure

The QOL is influenced by one's group membership. Primary group membership involves emotional connections, intimacy, and face-to-face interaction, such as the family, the playgroup, etc. One's primary group membership can be highly important and the basis of one's motivation. Secondary group relationships are relatively impersonal, based upon a common interest, such as a profession of carpenters, but with a low level of emotional involvement. Members of secondary groups need not be face-to-face. However, whether primary or secondary, groups have structure. That is, there are roles of leader and follower, individuals performing various functions such as record-keeper, critic, humorist, manager, etc.

Headaches

Husband–wife couples form a primary group. In this group, the QOL of one member is affected by the health status of the other. A group member cares about the well-being of the other member. Groot and van den Brink (2003) developed a model that accounts for these interdependencies. In it, they assume happiness to be determined by income, the presence of migraine headache in husband and wife, co-morbidity, and by other individual characteristics. Data from the October 1993, Dutch survey includes 4,700 households in which the head of the household is between 43 and 65 years of age. The life satisfaction of men and women in the survey is the same, but women tend to rate their life satisfaction slightly higher than men do (15.9 for men vs. 20.2 for women for the top-two life satisfaction options). Other studies show that migraine headaches affect women more than men, 6% of men and 15–17% women. Migraine is a debilitating condition, reducing one's QOL, limiting one's activities, bringing about sick leave and thereby reducing productivity, and reducing work capability. Substantial economic costs result from the condition. In the sample, 26% of women and 13% of men reported having suffered migraine during the past 12 months. These prevalences are slightly higher than rates for the general population, perhaps because of the slightly older age range of the sample. In the model, a number of household variables are controlled, as are other health conditions. The data of the model show that the presence of migraine reduces well-being. Findings show that the migraine has different effects on male and female. If the male partner has migraine, the well-being of the female partner is reduced. If the female partner has migraine, the husband is not similarly affected. Women, being more compassionate and empathetic, suffer for their partner. The study transformed the income variable to its log and found that life satisfaction increases with income. In another model, the presence of arthrosis of knees, hips, or hands of one partner adversely affects the life satisfaction of the other partner. Thus, the empathy of one partner for the other, in illness, negatively affects the other partner in husband–wife couples.

A six-grade class of a school in free-play recreation will form a structure that will include isolates, individuals who play alone. Identifying isolates, the teacher may influence playgroup structure by assigning the isolate to activities with individuals who rank high in the status in the group. Pre- and post-tests of self-concept and self-esteem will gauge the effect of the teacher's intervention. Alternately, a sociometric schedule may be administered to chart the social structure of the class and provide the teacher with the needed information for intervention to incorporate isolates into the group.

The same procedure may be followed with a teen-age sample, using rewards and other incentives to reorder the group structure and induce isolates into group participation with established leaders, as has been successfully done (Whyte, 1943).

The concept may be further explored by charting the sociometric relations in a neighborhood of families, and initiating interventions such as neighborhood parties, dinners, improvement programs, animal parades, and other such activities that stimulate participation. Before and after self-concept measures would provide evidence, along with subjective QOL measures. For a review of means of manipulation, see Nowak, Vollacher, and Miller, 2003.

The objective of this procedure is to encourage social inclusion and cohesion, by creating social support and thereby improving the individual's self-concept. Activities originating in primary and secondary groups impact the QOL.

Leisure Time

The constructive use of leisure time enhances the QOL. Constructive leisure time activities cultivate a positive self-concept, provide positive emotions, and enhance positive interpersonal relations with others. Fun in leisure activities, relaxation, enjoyment of physical and mental engagement, and creativity bring satisfaction and emotional rewards.

Yoshitaka Iwasaki (2007), in an extensive essay, identified pathways to leisure activities that affect the QOL. Positive emotions emerge from leisure activities such as hiking in the wilderness, building self-confidence through yoga or Tai Chi disciplines, or meditation: quietly contemplating the meaning of life. Leisure devoted to music, art, reading fiction, or constructing crafts builds one's self-esteem and self-identity. Leisure need not be spent alone. Activities with others in primary and secondary groups build social and cultural meanings that invoke satisfactions and spiritual experiences. Thus, positive emotions experienced in leisure activities benefit QOL.

Iwasaki (2007) quotes R.F. Baumeister's four "needs of meaning" that facilitate the quest for understanding life: (1) the need to have a purpose, connecting the present with the future; (2) the need for values to give goal-orientation to life; (3) the need for a sense of efficacy, the sense that one is important and can have an impact; (4) the need for a sense of self-worth, that one is worthy. Leisure provides the opportunity to satisfy these four needs and builds upon cultural means of satisfying them.

Constructive use of leisure time creates meanings that bring positive emotions and happiness. It facilitates contending with life's trials, what Shakespeare called "the heartache and thousand natural shocks that flesh is heir to." Giving meaning to life's leisure experiences is the key.

Leisure also provides a pathway to enhancing the QOL through using social means to contend with "the slings and arrows of outrageous fortune." Life's challenges are met through music, dance, storytelling, traditional rituals, and even humor and laughter. Following cultural prescriptions for dealing with difficulties leads to resolution of problems, and this is done through leisure activities. Individuals differ, depending upon their cultural orientation, and being loyal to their cultural mandates promotes satisfaction.

Throughout life, continuous development of interests and activities contributes to one's QOL. Through leisure activities, one learns and develops across the life span. Keiber, as quoted by Iwasaki (2007), identifies leisure's contributions to development, including becoming capable, secure, defining self in relation to others, continuing intimacy with others, playing a part of something bigger than oneself, and creating meaning.

Supreme Court Justice William O. Douglas extolled the benefits of a wilderness experience by saying the height is reached when one can whack a bear on the butt with a canoe paddle. People may find delight and satisfaction through other leisure-time adventures, as briefly outlined above, but the benefits to the QOL through constructive leisure activities is undeniable. Iwasaki (2007), to whom this author is indebted for the above ideas, presents examples and cross-cultural discussion of leisure.

This chapter has pointed to the importance to the QOL of becoming mentally healthy and developing self-assurance through leisure activities. Spiritual experiences provide reassurance and give life meaning. As a principal resource, one's primary group gives meaning, despite sometimes difficult family problems, such as teen pregnancy or child physical disfunctions, that test character and integrity. Friendship and neighborliness provide social support and satisfaction. Participation in group activities during leisure time, especially with in-group members, leads to gratification and enjoyment. Social inclusion diminishes isolation. Individuals who are involved create a positive, secure self-concept. Humankind strives also for mastery, to which we now turn.

Chapter 3
Mastery

Whatsoever thy hand findeth to do, do it with thy might; for
there is no work, nor device, nor knowledge, nor wisdom, in the
grave, whither thou goest.

Ecclesiastes 9:10

To admit poverty is no disgrace for a man; but, to make no effort to escape it is indeed disgraceful.

Thucydides (460–400 BC), Book 2

You must keep your goal in sight,
Labor toward it day and night,
Then at last arriving there –
You shall be too old to care.

–Witter Bynner, Wisdom

Mastery. Being successful, capable, ambitious, having a purpose in life, making a social contribution with aims and objectives in mind. In our civilization, the basis for mastery is found in the institutions of education and economy.

Proposition 3. The QOL may be enhanced by reducing income inequality, by minimizing other sources of differentiation, by augmenting successful outcomes to life's experiences in achieving life's goals, and by contributing to community civic and social life.

Free Markets

Fredrich August von Hayek, the Austrian economist who died in 1992, said the most efficient means of distributing goods and services was free-market capitalism (Cassidy, 2000). History is proving him correct. Free-market capitalism must be supported by norms and values of the culture. The essential values are respect for private property, the inviolability of contracts, and honesty in transactions. The free-market system falters when these three values are not respected. When these three values are violated – when private property is disregarded, when contracts are dishonored, when dishonesty enters into business transactions – the free-market system falters. But if the values are maintained, goods and services are produced,

A.L. Ferriss, *Approaches to Improving the Quality of Life*, Social Indicators Research
Series 42, DOI 10.1007/978-90-481-9148-2_3, © Springer Science+Business Media B.V. 2010

information is distributed, and needs are satisfied through buying and selling in the marketplace. Free-market capitalism predominates.

Because their values do not support a free market or their political organization prohibits it, many undeveloped societies cannot benefit from these principals. Corruption stymies enterprise in many countries. Growth is limited, owing to such depressive factors as corrupt administration in government and in enterprises, dictatorial dominance that obstructs an open system, and opposition to economic growth. The benefits of a free market are dissipated.

Economists point to the rise of the Industrial Revolution in England following 1800 through its system of open markets, low taxes, and a politically stable government. Middle-class values found support: "patience, hard work, ingenuity, innovativeness, education." To these advantages the sociologist Max Weber attributes the ethics of Protestantism, wherein hard work and thrift lead to success, a sign of God's favor.

Income inequality results from the industrial structure of the locality and the stage of the economy. The structure of industry may dictate a few highly paid technicians, as would be the case in computer manufacturing, or a large number of unskilled workers as in some production industries. Inequality of income in the United States has been rising since the 1970s. It has been increasing and the rate of increase has been rising. Authorities give reasons that include the decline in manufacturing jobs and the increasing proportion of service jobs which pay less. In addition, the number of females in the labor force has increased, with females typically working in lower paying jobs. The percent of households headed by a female has increased. Inequality of income, in a study of US counties, is negatively associated with percent of females employed and positively associated with percent of female heads of households (Albrecht & Albrecht, 2007). The trend in inequality may be countered through improving skills through education and training and through installing economic enterprises that employ skilled employees.

Females have increased in the labor force. Their earnings, being typically lower, have lead to increased income inequality. However, a recent study by Albrecht (2007), using more than 3,000 US counties in the analysis, demonstrated that social conditions of the county (that is, the demographic and family composition and related factors) influence inequality more than economic conditions. Albrecht showed that female employment, in contributing to family income, lowers income inequality. The presence of female-headed households increases inequality. Inequality of income affects the QOL of a community when it results in greater poverty and larger numbers of low-income families. This trend may be countered through education and training and development of businesses that employ skilled labor.

Income

Per capita income has been the bellwether of QOL discussions, because income enables purchase of items that satisfy needs. Some have said that the more income one has, the better the QOL. This is false. As discussed in Chapter 4 in connection with happiness, as the per capita income increases up to the point where basic needs – clothing, shelter, food – are met, the QOL also rises. Beyond this point, increases in income have but small impact on the QOL. Refer to the discussion in Chapter 4.

Some light is cast on this problem by an economic study. Three indicators are used by Mazumdar (2000) to reflect the QOL: life expectancy at birth, infant survival rate, and adult literacy rate. She divided countries of the world into three groups: 20 high-income countries, 40 middle-income countries, and 32 low-income countries. Using a lagged dependent variable model, she regressed the well-being indices, taken together and taken separately. For the high-income group of countries, she found per capita income and well-being to be independent of each other. For the middle- and low-income countries, she found a "causal flow" between the well-being indices and per capita income up to a certain level of income. However, beyond this "certain minimum level" of per capita income, the two (well-being and per capita income) are independent of each other. Where the level of social development is low, well-being indicators also are low. Low development is implied by "undeveloped infra-structure and low labour productivity which in turn implies low per capita real gross domestic product." She states that this is a "typical vicious cycle phenomenon." Time wise, life expectancy at birth and infant survival rate precede an increase in per capita income, while the adult literacy rate follows per capita income improvement. These results are important for structuring growth of less developed countries, as well as for the improvement of QOL.

Success

Achieving success in one's work requires dedicated effort, long working hours beyond the normal daily grind, and sacrifices of other life activities. A person's devotion to an occupation eliminates many of the pleasures and amenities of normal living. Studies show that such devotion to work often removes the worker from the family and leads to neglect of family relationships. The result, however, is recognition of accomplishments, perhaps financial security, and the satisfaction of achieving a goal. One ambitious for success should be aware of this price to pay for mastery. Steps can be taken to minimize these unwanted consequences. "Quality time" with family members could be scheduled. Where appropriate, some family members might be involved in the work of the breadwinner. If financial benefits accompany success, extending such benefits to family members in the form perhaps of trips, recreation equipment, and other amenities would compensate for the breadwinner's absence. With mastery achieved, the breadwinner may devote more than normal time to family relationships, thereby enhancing better QOL.

Sirgy, Reilly, Wu, and Efraty (2008) developed a model relating the quality of work life with the QOL. They theorized that the following aspects of work life influence the QOL: "(1) providing appropriate work resources to meet the expectations of employee role identities, (2) reducing role conflict in work and non-work life, (3) enhancing multiple role identities, (4) reducing role demands, (5) reducing stress related to work and non-work role identities, and (6) increasing the value of role identity." They theorized that a variety of work-life conditions and a variety of home conditions, taken together with the quality of work life, serve to enhance the QOL. They propose continued research on these dimensions.

Poverty

Worldwide poverty presents a major international problem, its chief monitor being the World Bank. In 2007, it announced that 985 million people were living in poverty, a reduction from 1990 of 260 million. The Bank defines poverty as a person living daily on the local equivalent in 1993 of $1.08 for the purchase of food. Economists criticize the World Bank's method of estimating world poverty. Critics say that by increasing the estimate of the cost of a day's sustenance to $1.22, the estimate of world poverty increases to 1.37 billion, about 23% of the world population. Climatic differences, errors in national surveys, food costs, and other factors render international estimates unreliable. Poverty, however, is a major international problem, a critical source of friction between have and have-not nations. Its solution rests upon increasing the production of wealth in a country and distributing income more equitably. Production of wealth is the key to reducing poverty (Moss, 1999).

A Canadian study of time-deprived poverty-level people found two-thirds of the population of more than 2,200 sample respondents neither time nor money-poor. Only 5% were both time and money-poor. About one-fifth of the sample was time-poor but not money-poor. In summary, about one-fourth were time-poor, meaning that they felt a deficit in discretionary time to devote to their family and other outside activities (Harvey & Mukhopadhyay, 2007). How important to QOL is discretionary time with the family?

In countries where there is excess labor force, more workers than the economy requires, migration becomes a possible solution. By removing the unemployed from the area, the percentage employed increases and a more satisfactory average QOL results. The migrants to another country, likewise, stand a chance in their new country of employment and improving their QOL. In recent history, Germany employed immigrants to bolster its labor force. A recent study of migration from Ghana and Egypt (Sabates-Wheeler, Sabates, & Castaldo, 2008) shows the moderating effects of migration on poverty in those countries. "(I)mmigration offers a better chance of breaking through persistent poverty." For best results, the migrants should be guided to countries with employment opportunities, a process difficult to impose in open societies.

Based upon Australian data, Headey (2008) has devised a more inclusive definition of poverty. To the usual income, he also includes consumption practice and wealth. When the three measures are used, the percent in poverty is greatly reduced in Australia.

Child Poverty

Child poverty creates stress in the child's life. According to Gary W. Evans, ecologist at Cornell University, stress leads to poor memory, which is critical in learning. Child poverty is a critical indicator of the QOL. A study of child poverty in the 159 counties of Georgia, USA (Ferriss, 2006), identified the structure of the county as associated with child poverty. A factor analysis of these county characteristics resulted in three types of counties: "deprived/rural" counties harbored child poverty, while child poverty was minimal in counties identified as "business/money" and "progressive/urban." Structural features of the county were positively associated with child poverty: residential stability, unemployment, low educational achievement, youth and age dependency, single parent female household heads with children, grandparent child care, and health disability of child, elders, and of working age persons. Structural features militating against child poverty were persons with more education than average, higher population density, higher out-migration, a population of largely married families, one with higher retail sales in dollar value, a large middle class, higher weekly wages, and other minor structural features. The study found that child poverty levels differed in counties with largely black children in poverty from those with largely white children in poverty. The study concluded that intervention to reduce child poverty should address the two sets of counties differently.

While this study used the Federal definition of a family in poverty as identifying child poverty, Moore, Vandivere, and Redd (2006) have refined an index of children at risk. Called a Sociodemographic Risk Index, it consists of five variables: family income, family structure, parent education, family size, and home ownership. From 0 to 5, the Risk Index classifies children in terms of the number of risk factors present. For 1997 and 1999 data from the National Survey of American Families, 17.5% of children were subject to three or more risk factors. This compares with 17.1% of children in poverty (2005) according to Census definition. The Sociodemographic Risk Index for children provides a useful analytical tool for monitoring the status of children and for identifying characteristics associated with the Index.

The problem of poverty is at the heart of world progress. Why have European, Western, and a few other nations (e.g., Japan, Hong Kong) developed economically, creating wealth, while many others have remained traditional and largely undeveloped? Some see the answer in the cultural practices of the country. Changing such cultural norms is one key to stimulating economic action.

Developing small-scale enterprises that produce commodities and provide services is a key to erasing poverty in third-world countries, according to a theory expounded by Samli (2008). He advocates a bottoms-up approach. Developing third-world countries' economies by promoting such entrepreneurs will "enhance the social health and environmental well-being" according to Samli. He decries the fact that in a number of African countries, many businesses are owned and operated by the government, thereby nullifying the creation of small enterprises. His suggestion is consistent with the experience of small-scale enterprises encouraged through small-scale loans, described below.

The discussion of poverty is continued in Chapter 7, Conservatism.

Materialism

Materialism is defined as devotion to material things, as opposed to spiritual, and is characterized by consumerism. Paradoxically, studies have found materialism inversely related to QOL. Even with gender, education, age, and income held constant, materialism remains negatively correlated with QOL. Persons devoted to extrinsic goals, that is, goals dependent upon external rewards, tend to a lower QOL. When persons set high standards of living that cannot be met, they are dissatisfied with their QOL. Roberts and Clement (2007) cite a number of studies that support the hypothesis that material values and materialism are negatively associated with QOL. Consequently, as one strives for mastery, one should not seek for material objects and benefits. This is consistent with some religious beliefs. For example, Hindu philosophy holds that one should not strive for the results of action.

Religion

Faith-based organizations, religious denominations, with sympathy for the mis-begotten, the poor, and the needy, have extended their helping hands throughout the world. As an example, The Millennium Development Goals of the Episcopal Church include eight objectives: eradicate extreme poverty and hunger, achieve universal primary education for children, promote gender equality and empower women, reduce child mortality, improve mental health, combat HIV/AIDS, malaria, and other diseases, ensure environmental sustainability, and create a global partnership for development. They set the target year for these objectives at 2015. In the face of these noble goals, the efforts seem meager, indeed, but small gains do accumulate. One set of programs, for example, created a school lunch program in Haiti, strengthened a primary school in Ecuador, and built classrooms for girls in Tanganyika. A team each year provides medical care to a group in Honduras, helped open a maternity clinic in Dar es Salaam, Tanzania, and distributes mosquito nets and blankets. The program links individual US churches with the foreign activity. These are only samples of the many such efforts that religious organizations sponsor, support, and promote. The motivation rests upon the denomination's goal of relieving the suffering of human kind (Shew, 2007). Such efforts enhance the QOL in many ways.

Small Business Loans

The Foundation for International Community Assistance (FINCA) promotes small-enterprise business loans as a step in reducing global poverty. Based in Washington, DC, FINCA sponsors village banks. These banks are managed by local people to provide small loans (up to $500) to local entrepreneurs. "They choose their investments, disburse and collect all loans, manage their savings, elect their officers, write their by-laws, and keep their books." They do this to provide low-interest loans to poor people who could not qualify for a normal bank loan. Self-employment loans enable the poor to establish money-yielding activities within their capabilities. Loans have been used for establishing retail stores, manufacturing bricks, raising chickens or pigs, baking bread for sale, knitting sweaters, starting a handicraft, and the like. When loans are repaid, the person is eligible for new loans. Records show that 95% of the loans are repaid. Local people manage the village bank, know the recipient of the loan, and see that the loan is repaid, the secret of the program's success. Thus, enterprise based upon individual initiative, rather than gifts, provides a means out of poverty, especially for women. They gain independence and improve their QOL. The concept of microfinance programs was originated some years ago by the Ford Foundation in India.

BRAC – Building Resources Across Communities – was founded by Fazie Hasan Abed. It has a staff of over 125,000 that have issued over $5.5 billion in small loans of $100–200. It has helped nearly 7 million poor women. Small loans have been repaid at the rate of 98.7%. Begun in the 1970s in Bangladesh, BRAC has transformed the lives of millions through its anti-poverty work. In addition to the microfinance program, it trains health workers who go door to door, educating householders in health practices and preventive measures for malaria, tuberculosis, and other common diseases. BRAC also trains teachers and operates 53,000 pre-primary and primary schools. Over 6 million children have passed through its schools. Its graduates then go on to secondary schools in large numbers. In 2008, BRAC was awarded the Conrad N. Hilton Humanitarian Prize for its multifaceted approach to relieving poverty. In addition to Bangladesh, it works in Liberia, Pakistan, Sierra Leone, Southern Sudan, Sri Lanka, Tanzania, and Uganda. For developing countries of Asia and Africa, the program offers a road out of poverty and a chance for a better QOL.

Employment

Most countries are experiencing transitions in the combination of occupations that compose their labor force. They are finding an increase in knowledge-based jobs. In striving to remain competitive, European countries, at a Lisbon meeting of the European Council in 2000, outlined four strategies as follows: "(a) reaching a knowledge-based economy; (b) modernizing the European social model; (c) developing a framework of appropriate and stability-oriented macroeconomic policies; (d) achieving sustainable development." To these high objectives, the European Council in 2005 identified three specific objectives, namely (a) "more and better jobs for Europe: developing an active employment policy." This would include "improving employability and reducing skill gaps; increasing adaptability through lifelong learning; increasing employment in services; and reducing occupational segregation." (b) "Education and training for living and working in the knowledge society." This includes such things as developing learning centers that would promote learning new skills. (c) "Promoting Social Inclusion" (Royuela, Lopez-Tamayo, & Surinach, 2008). These objectives would apply to any country having an interest in improving the employability of its citizens in order to improve the quality of work life (QWL).

A study of Finland's unemployment in the years 1990, 1996, and 2000 inquired into the consequences of unemployment on happiness and subjective well-being (Bockerman & Ilmakunnas, 2006). The data were from the World Values Survey. During the early 1990s, unemployment increased, but subjective well-being did not decline. Unemployment is not related to life satisfaction and happiness in Finland. Unemployment affects the movement from low to high happiness, but at high happiness levels, unemployment is insignificant. Perhaps the welfare system provides the security that underlies this result.

Summary of Initiatives

Under a free-market economic system, one may gain mastery through education free enterprise and through applying one's talents. Several devices may stimulate effort: low-interest loans through village banks, assistance through gifts from faith-based organizations and Heifer International to start enterprises, and factories that create goods to satisfy needs and augment the QOL. BRAC works in areas of Africa and Asia to bring keys to the door out of poverty. These initiatives have proven successful. Corruption countermands these efforts in many less developed countries. The norms of free-market capitalism – private property, secure contracts, and honesty – need to be instilled and practiced (Land, 2005) and (Kahneman et al. 2004).

Income inequality may be a fact of life. However, those occupying the lower rungs of income should earn enough for a satisfactory QOL. This may require that persons in the middle and upper levels of income transfer income to the lowest levels. Norms and values to support such income distribution need to be established by governments. Some welfare-state European countries have approached this ideal, notably Denmark.

Thus, the economic system, as influenced by the education and political system, is the basis for improving the mastery aspect of QOL.

National initiatives are needed to improve the quality of work life, following the specifics set forth by the European Commission, to create more jobs, train for new jobs in a knowledge-based society, and promote social inclusion.

Chapter 4
Affective Autonomy

The things which ... are esteemed as the greatest good of all,
... can be reduced to these three headings: to wit, Riches, Fame,
and Pleasure. With these three the mind is so engrossed that it
cannot scarcely think of any other good.
      Benedict Spinoza, Tractatus de Intellectus Emendatione
      (1677) 1, 3.

The best portion of a good man's life,–
His little, nameless, unremembered acts
Of kindness and love.
      –*William Wordsworth, Lines Composed a Few Miles Above*
      Tintern Abbey.

The thing that numbs the heart is this:
That men cannot devise
Some scheme of life to banish fear
That lurks in most men's eyes.
                                          –James Norman Hall, Fear

Affective Autonomy. Having pleasure, enjoying an exciting life, emotional well-being. These good things come to us during our leisure hours, identified as recreational activities. Low affective autonomy is characterized by concern with others' evaluations of self and their expectations and unhappiness.

Proposition 4. The QOL may be enhanced by removing the reasons for depression, suicide, and other negative responses, and by experiencing pleasure and an exciting life, through love, affection, and emotional well-being.

These good things come to us during our leisure hours – recreational activities. Low affective autonomy is characterized by concern with others' evaluations of self and destructive use of leisure time. A key to enhancing affective autonomy lies in expanding the constructive use of leisure time, filled with pleasurable leisure experiences, and building bases for happiness.

As we interact with others in groups, we may run the gamut of positive or negative emotions. Positive emotions include joy, happiness, love, etc., while negative emotions may be sadness, fear, anger, etc. We will have a more desirable and satisfying QOL by maximizing positive emotions (Grigg, 1996).

A.L. Ferriss, *Approaches to Improving the Quality of Life*, Social Indicators Research   29
Series 42, DOI 10.1007/978-90-481-9148-2_4, © Springer Science+Business Media B.V. 2010

A German psychological study has identified two components of subjective well-being (Schimmack et al., 2008): affective well-being and cognitive well-being. In the present study, Affective Autonomy and Intellectual Autonomy are treated as independent domains. The German study found that research findings for the affective component were not duplicated for the cognitive component, showing that the two are independent domains. Consequently, efforts to improve the two need to be separate and independent.

Role Behavior

Role Conflict

We play many roles. Playing them well may augment one's QOL. One role usually dominates: mother, worker, professional, son, etc., but we need to be prepared also to meet the requirements of several roles. The demands of one role may conflict with those of another, creating emotional problems. For example, the demands of job may conflict with the needs of the role in the family. This may be especially the case among females who have a professional role, a mother role, and the duties of a wife. As another example, a religious adherent may subscribe to ethical principles that cannot be practiced in his business role.

Some role requirements may specify emotional restrictions, autonomy being minimized. For example, the clerk in a merchandise store must control his/her anger in the face of disparagement by a customer, as "The customer is always right." The clerk must exercise emotional discipline, suppressing a defensive retort. One must adapt to such role requirements if one is to enjoy a satisfying QOL.

Emotion

Research has identified emotional conditions that accompany a better QOL. Women, more than men, experience negative emotions. The unmarried, more than married persons, and the less educated, more than the more educated, frequently experience distress. The birth of a child affects the emotional state of a family, initially creating negative emotions that eventually change as the family adjusts to the new member. Strong religious faith accompanies positive emotions. Undesirable life events, such as the death of a loved one, result in negative emotions. Over the life course, emotional status typically changes: youth and middle-aged persons are more depressed, the condition declining to about age 55 years and then turning negative again. These are observations from surveys of emotion. Cultural conditions affect emotions, and they may not hold in all social situations (Wisecup, Robinson, & Smith-Lovin, 2007). In fact, some studies have shown older people to be less, rather than more, depressed than those of younger ages. One needs the confidence of positive emotions – joy, love, happiness – for a satisfying QOL.

The emotion of loneliness was found associated with seven domains of a life satisfaction scale in two communities in Australia (Bramston et al., 2002). Lonely people reported consistently lower QOL. A Neighborhood Cohesion measure of the community was not associated with subjective well-being. The authors reasoned that the QOL would improve when intervention reduced the basis for loneliness. The QOL domains were material, health, learning, intimacy, safety, community, and emotion, as measured by the Cummins-Cahill scale.

Income and Happiness

Has the enormous improvement in wealth of most countries' economies over the last several decades increased happiness? The question raises questions. The economist Richard A. Easterlin (1974) presents evidence that, in many countries, the increase in national per capita income has not improved average happiness. It is called "The Easterlin paradox." Hagerty and Veenhoven (2003, 2006), on the other hand, present evidence which they state demonstrates that happiness increases with the corresponding improvement in per capita income. "The results show that increasing national income does go with increasing national happiness." Data for 21 countries are examined, seven showing a positive relationship with growth and happiness. A recent study in SINET, November 2009, by Diener and Kaheneman, concluded that economic growth affects some but not all types of SWB. They conclude that more research is needed on how societies influence negative and positive emotions, which is also a contention of this book.

In their 2003 paper, Hagerty and Veenhoven present graphs of the US data based upon a four-step happiness scale that is level, with no visible slope over time. They also show a happiness scale from the US General Social Survey, showing a flat regression over time. However, when the question asked respondents is not "How happy are you?" but Cantril's Worst-Best Possible Life, and the Gallup's life satisfaction scale of US samples, a slight increase is observed. Average happiness in western Europe tapped by the *Eurobarometer* reveals a slight increase. A sample of other nations over varying periods also shows increases.

Subjective well-being in Japan, over time (1958–2007), with 42 observations, revealed a modest but significant relationship with Japan real GDP per capita (Suzuki, 2009). The author thinks that the Japanese people lost confidence in the economic system in the late 1990s, and this may have influenced their opinions.

It appears that the use of a question other than straightforward "happiness" reveals an increase over time, while the use of the "happiness" question does not. In any case, the increase in happiness and life satisfaction is very slight when compared with the increase in per capita income or per capita GDP. "The Easterlin paradox" can now be examined with more definitive data.

In a study using data from the World Values Survey involving 43 countries, the authors found that increases in both relative and absolute income prompted increases in happiness. Changes in relative income were more important in influencing happiness than changes in absolute income. However, the authors found that non-income factors influenced happiness to a greater extent than income: such factors as health, marital status, and employment/unemployment (Ball & Chernova, 2008).

An increase in family income up to a point goes with an increase in happiness and life satisfaction, but beyond that point, an increase in income has little effect. A study of nine European nations by Seghieri et al. (2006) essentially confirms this result. They state, "... (A)lthough the rich are typically more satisfied with their financial situation than the poor, this happens only up to a point." And, "... (I)ndividual and environmental characteristics influence subjective satisfaction at least as much as, and possibly more than, income."

Haller and Handler (2006) used the World Values Survey, 1995–1997, to study happiness and life satisfaction in 41 countries. They report the same exponential curve of per capita GNP and life satisfaction, as described above (Seghieri et al., 2006). An increase in per capita income increases life satisfaction up to a point (in this case between 10,000 and 20,000 per capita), but beyond that point, increases in per capita income have little effect upon life satisfaction. The authors also show a strong national linear relationship between life satisfaction and happiness but do not report the value of the correlation coefficient.

National Income and Happiness

As per capita income of nations increases, happiness and life satisfaction increase – up to a certain income level. This income level possibly is the point that basic needs are satisfied. At this point, discretionary income becomes available to the average household. Beyond this point, an increase in income prompts only a slight increase in happiness and life satisfaction. The evidence relies upon the average of nations and is presented in Veenhoven (1993) and in Ferriss (1999). Recently, a study showed that spending money for gifts to others is more likely to foster one's happiness than spending it on one's self. This result also was found for 41 countries of the World Values Survey, 1995–1997, by Haller and Hadler (2006), as reported previously.

Happiness Concisely Considered

Accepting the Easterlin paradox, the Dalai Lama's, Buddhist's, and others' positions, we conclude that happiness is a mind-set, an attitude, a "way we see." As a subjective expression of well-being, "... happiness and joy are understood to be a function of a tamed and disciplined mind." Tranquility of mind and our attitudes toward "things" should be positive. But how does the mind get that way? According to many cited above, the mind reacts to external situations, family, friends, and community. A person must be virtuous and devoted to a divine spirit. One does not work for happiness. One gains happiness by attending to the happiness of others, not one's own happiness. Some say feeling good and enjoying life is important, others point to being unhappy occasionally, so that when happiness comes, we appreciate it. More money, once there is enough for the essentials, does not bring happiness – only if a person is in dire need does money help. Those are the diverse and manifold concepts of happiness. Which we accept may depend upon our age, or our society, or our culture. In any event, people are motivated to achieve it. It is a prime indicator of SWB and QOL.

Emotional well-being leads to happiness. In fact, positive emotion *is* happiness. Our conception of it and our understanding of happiness are affected by our culture and our social situation.

Aristotle wrote, "If happiness is activity in accordance with excellence, it is reasonable that it should be in accordance with the highest excellence." "Excellence" depends upon cultural values that define excellence. He also wrote in his *Ethics*, "Happiness depends upon ourselves." Others have added that our relations with others are critical. Thus, our social life influences our happiness.

Ricard (2000) also pointed to the road to happiness: "Happiness is the result of inner maturity. It depends on us alone, and requires patient work, carried out from day to day. Happiness must be built, and this requires time and effort. In the long run, happiness and unhappiness are therefore a way of being, a life skill." Cicero, in his *De Natura Deorum,* took the thought a step further: "A happy life consists of tranquility of mind."

> Happiness is the main object of our aspirations, whatever name we give to it: fulfillment, deep satisfaction, serenity, accomplishment, wisdom, fortune, joy or inner peace, and however we try to seek it: creativity, justice, altruism, striving, competition of a plan or a piece of work (Ricard, 2000).

A recent study (Headey, 2008) found that life satisfaction is promoted when one's goals involve family, friends, and the community, but not when one's goals center upon materialism and career success. A study of 34 years of the General Social Survey concluded that people are happier who are active in social affairs, religion, and reading newspapers, but not in TV viewing (Robinson & Martin, 2008).

Positive thinking provides a mode for achieving happiness. The Roman Emperor Marcus Aurelius wrote that happiness "depends upon the quality of your thoughts." How one reacts to events and interprets them in the mind, whether positively or negatively, determines the effect of the event upon our psychological mind-set. The positive reaction is more likely to result in happy demeanor. Leo Tolstoy concurs: "Happiness does not depend upon outward things, but on the way we see them." The primacy of a positive reaction in generating happiness is also advanced by Forni (2002). "So by happiness I mean feeling good – enjoying life and wanting the feeling to be maintained" (Layard, 2005).

Buddhist culture centers upon compassion for others and happiness as an objective of life. The 14th Dalai Lama concurs in the basis of happiness, saying: "Right now, at this very moment, we have a mind which is all the basic equipment we need to achieve complete happiness" (Dalai Lama & Cutler, 1999). It is all in the mind, but striving for something other than happiness may be the key to finding happiness.

Religion offers devotion to the divine spirit as the key to happiness. For example, the Hebrew Bible, Psalm 84:

> ".... O Lord of hosts, my King and my God,
> 3. Happy are they who dwell in your house!
>   They will always be praising you.
> 4. Happy are the people whose strength is in you!
>   Whose hearts are set on the pilgrims' way."

John Stuart Mill said it this way: "Those only are happy who have their minds fixed on some object other than their own happiness; on the happiness of others, on the improvement of mankind, even on some art or pursuit, followed not as a means, but as itself an ideal end. Aiming thus at something else, they find happiness by the way", as quoted by Bornstein (2007).

An extensive study of happiness of Koreans (Kim et al., 2007) identified 16 factors they found to be essential for their happiness. Money ranked number six of the 16, reflecting a cultural value. Interpersonal relations, especially concerning children, ranked high. The 16 factors, separated into three domains, are as follows:

Intrapersonal factors: self-assurance, personal growth, autonomy, positive attitude, and religion.
Interpersonal factors: helping others, relationship with children, relationship with parents and siblings, intimate relationships, and relationship with others.
Living condition factors include money, leisure, social status, social environment, appearance, and health.

Kim et al. (2007) point out that age and cultural values affect the selection of factors that the Korean people identify as important for their happiness. Members of Asian culture are more likely to emphasize interpersonal relations, relationship with children, and religion than would representatives of Western culture.

Koreans (a collectivist society) and Japanese were compared with Canadians, an individualistic society, by Lee et al. (2000). The study concluded that, despite some cultural differences, the respondents employed the same understandings of happiness. Asian students, however, score lower on happiness than do the Canadian sample.

Of this mire of orientations, psychologists have identified *pleasure, engagement,* and *meaning* as the critical elements in happiness (Vella-Brodrick et al., 2009). These three best predict subjective well-being, but meaning and engagement together predict the greater variance in subjective well-being. This concurs with the eudaimonic concept of happiness that includes "personal growth, meaning, and serving a higher purpose" as the basis for achieving happiness. This is superior to the hedonic notion that pleasure is the pathway to happiness. In the Australian sample of the study, personality factors were included. It showed that extraversion was highly correlated with happiness, and its component, pleasure. These are psychological orientations and they rest, eventually, upon the socio-cultural content within which the individual interacts and finds meaning and satisfaction.

In keeping with the preceding observations, Haller and Hadler (2006) found support in data from the World Values Survey for four of their hypotheses. Happiness, they found, is a stable trait of individuals, characterized by positive and close social relationships. It is a consequence of one's objective life situation, characterized best by marriage and the family. They report the finding that the economic utility function of individuals is consistent with happiness. Consumer behavior reflects the tastes of individuals, the real well-being (utility). They emphasize the importance of participation in organizations, such as the religious. They also found support for the comparison hypothesis that people are satisfied when they find their own situation as well-off or better than others in their social class. They emphasize the importance to happiness of maintaining social relations and networks with other people. Working and living for others is the key. Happiness and satisfaction was also affected by the prosperous economic time of the 1990s, but countries in the former communist block, making the transition to a market economy, exerted a negative impact, more on the lower classes than on the middle classes. However, more developed countries improved the situation of the lower classes because of the general increase in wealth.

The general finding of the study is that life satisfaction and happiness arise from the interaction of individual characteristics, their aspirations and expectations, and the social relations and social structure in which they live. This reinforces the essential thesis of this book, namely that the social structure of the society exerts a definitive impact upon the QOL.

GSS Happiness

Employing the three-step General Social Survey item on happiness – "very," "pretty," and "not so" – Ferriss (1999) found the trend, 1972–1996, of the three items to present different inclines. The "not too happy" responses were generally flat but increased slightly during the period of decline in median family income of the early 1980s. At the other extreme, the "very happy" responses drift slightly downward during the period, ending about 5% points lower in 1996 than in 1972. This trend is negatively associated with median family income, $r = -17$. One might expect the "very happy" responses to increase with the slight increase in median family income, but such is not the case. The reason may be that people consider themselves "pretty happy," for that response, while volatile, showed the greatest increase, ending about 10% points higher in 1996 than its lowest point in 1975. However, if the "very happy" and the "pretty happy" responses are added together, they are correlated with median family income, income and happiness having 25% common variance. We conclude from this study that the trend in overall happiness is correlated with median family income in the United States during 1972–1996. A recent comparison of data from Australia, Britain, Germany, Hungary, and The Netherlands found that wealth affects happiness more than income, showing the importance of economic well-being (Headey et al., 2008).

Age and Happiness

Recent studies from the General Social Survey trace happiness by age. Older adults are found to be happier than the young. While older people reported more health problems than the young, they reported fewer overall difficulties, such as financial or crime problems. These results are consistent with the finding that older persons experience less depression than the middle-aged. The Survey also shows that those who work after age 65 report higher job satisfaction than younger workers. Older persons have more positive emotions and are more passive, emotionally. The Survey show young people experiencing anger, anxiety, and depression at higher levels than the middle-aged. The depression finding is contrary to another study that shows middle-aged persons to have higher depression, but the method of defining depression may be different. It has been observed that the well-being of older adults in the United States improved when social security payments to them began in the late 1930s. Energetic, pleasurable activities for older adults will elevate positive emotions and counteract loneliness, sadness, and depression.

Some of the above generalizations are supported by a study of 2,475 Taiwanese, aged 20 and older, in 1998 (Chen, 2003). The sample was divided for comparison into three age groups: up to 30, 30–59, and 60 and older. It found that the determinants of life satisfaction differ for these three groups. The life satisfaction of the elderly was influenced by financial status and the availability of financial support. The younger group, on the other hand, was influenced by not only financial status but also concern for leisure time activities and transportation. This group, of course, was beginning life and work careers, while the older group looked back upon a life of work. The life satisfaction of the middle-age group, on the other hand, was affected by most all life domains, except public safety. It was particularly affected by social changes. The authors viewed the older group as "retreating from society." While global life satisfaction here may be assumed to stand in for happiness, it is not quite the same. We may conclude that the uncertain financial status of elderly Taiwanese prompted their anxiety. In countries with stronger social security system for retirees, this would not be a major concern. From other sources, we find that the life expectancy in Taiwan is 75 years, the same as Denmark. On this measure, the country stands well with other nations that have high QOL.

Opinions/Attitudes

Affective autonomy and intellectual autonomy require the free expression of opinion. Opinion differences may cause friction between group members and adversely affect the QOL. When differences of opinion exist within the family, members need to discuss the problem calmly, so as to identify the bases of disagreement and come to equitable understandings, if not complete agreement, on the issues. Techniques of achieving such understandings have been devised under the heading, "conflict resolution" (q.v., Chapter 5).

Our attitudes are mental dispositions that influence our behavior. They may be positive or negative, favorable or unfavorable responses to an object, person, institution or event. These mental dispositions rest upon the values acquired through interaction with others in the family and other associates. When a group includes members with attitudes toward an important matter different from the others, a change of attitude may improve the consensus of the group. Psychologists have experimented with techniques for changing attitudes. While the character of the disagreement and the structure of the group may influence the most appropriate technique for attitude change, the following procedures have been shown to change attitudes:

(1) Present the person with information, which implies an attitude different from the one held by the person. If the person accepts the information, change in beliefs and attitude should result (Eagly, 2000).
(2) The person's beliefs about the object have consequences for the person's behavior and attitude toward the object. Someone considered to be an "expert" may persuade with conviction. The expert's credibility carries influence. Thus, confidence in the communicator is critical and leads to attitude change.

Belief in various social axioms, stereotypic folk values about social relations, impact self-esteem and life satisfaction. A study of Chinese students in Hong Kong illustrates the relationship. A cynical belief, for example, "Kind hearted people usually suffer losses," is negatively correlated with self-esteem and life satisfaction. The authors (Lai et al., 2007) conclude that beliefs about the world affect social experience and impact self-esteem. In turn, self-esteem promotes life satisfaction and well-being. The five social axioms in the study, taken together in a regression analysis, significantly predicted life satisfaction, $R^2 = 0.26$. The authors recommend that therapists identify a patient's beliefs and attempt to turn negative orientations into positive ones in the interest of improving self-esteem and life satisfaction.

Life satisfaction and QOL of the young (ages 15–29) of 21 European countries and Israel were compared with those of persons older than 30 years (Pichler, 2006). Questions on life satisfaction and happiness show that the young are happier than those older than 30 years. Thirty percent of the young report very high levels of QOL, while 26% reported low QOL. The young are happier and more satisfied with their lives than those older in Europe, according to the European Social Survey, round one. The young in Scandinavian countries (Denmark, Finland, Sweden, Norway) are the happiest, 50% ranking high or very high. Next most happy group are Central Europeans, with the young of Switzerland and Austria reaching 40% in high QOL. Among German young people, however, only 31% of them are in the high-QOL classification. Lower QOL is found among eastern and southern European youth, being around 30% or less. The author points to the reason for the youths' QOL as based upon their objective living conditions and "embeddedness" in society. "People with large social, political, and 'financial participatory' capital are more embedded in society and have not to fear social exclusion" (p. 429). Social capital is another term Pichler uses to explain embeddedness. His general conclusion reaffirms the position of the young in European society as willing to volunteer and participate in European life.

Values and QOL

One's opinions and attitudes rest heavily upon one's values. Values concerning the family include life satisfaction. In a study of Singaporeans, Tan (2006) found that family values contributed strongly to satisfaction with life and social well-being. The measure of family values consisted of an eight-item scale related to nurturing and upholding family values. Values, identifying what are good and desirable, are derived from our cultural milieu in which the family institution is primary. Next, the character of associations in the neighborhood is included, followed by interaction with others in the community, for children, the school, especially. Acquisition of values is largely unconscious.

The European Social Survey (ESS), initiated in 2002 with surveys every other year, now provides data for examining well-being in relation to the various cultures: east Europe, west Europe, Scandinavia, southern Europe. European social scientists have taken advantage of the opportunity ESS offers and produced hundreds of analyses, especially of life satisfaction in relation to other influences.

Georgellis and associates (2009), using the first two rounds of ESS, have reinforced the finding that life satisfaction is positively related to income. However, when the respondent compares his/her income with that of others in the same educational category – reference income – life satisfaction and income are negatively associated. The study finds that personal values and beliefs exert a strong influence on life satisfaction. Differences in values are evident in international comparisons. Religious influences in western and southern Europe positively affect life satisfaction, whereas this is not the finding for Scandinavia. Being creative in western and southern Europe exerts a positive effect on life satisfaction, but not in Scandinavia. Materialism is an interesting value. Studies have shown it negatively associated with happiness and life satisfaction. This study also found this true for western Europe and Scandinavia, but not for southern Europe, where materialism is associated with higher life satisfaction. Values and beliefs, thus, are powerful influences. As Robert Browning, the English poet, commenting on the variety of beliefs, wrote:

> While I watched my foolish heart expand
> In the lazy glow of benevolence,
> O'er the various modes of man's belief.

Motivation

The change agent also must consider motivation to change. The communicator should couch persuasive statements to motivate the target person. If the spread between the target's current attitude and the one desired by the communicator is considerable, resistance to change can arise. A strategy for overcoming such resistance should be devised based upon the validity of belief of the target person, for beliefs underlie attitudes.

An attitude may be changed through acting out behavior that is consistent with the changed attitude. The target person is placed in a role where he/she acts out the behavior reflecting the attitude. Behavior consistent with a changed attitude stimulates acceptance of that attitude. This is a powerful approach to attitude change (Eagly, 2000). In applying role-playing, the target person's identity must be considered, so that the integrity of the role-player is not violated. The role-player must accept the idea of the role, assuming that the behavior is consistent with the desired attitude.

In addition to role-playing, restructuring the life situation of the target person can be effective, especially if restructuring satisfies motivational interests of the target. Both strategies can lead to attitude change in cases where such change would improve the QOL.

Most behavior is goal directed. Goals represent some culture value. One's attitudes should be consistent with the value. If they are inconsistent, cognitive dissonance arises, which may lead to psychic conflict. But when attitudes are consistent with the goal-directed value, the person achieves an effective level of motivation. Some psychological studies have shown a weak relationship between attitudes and values (Prentice, 2000). However, consistency between goals, values, and attitudes leads to personal integrity.

The National Mood

Affective relations are influenced by the national mood, currently (2009) one of anxiety over the possibility of terrorist attack. Fear, sometimes violent, is an emotional reaction to a threat, real or imagined. Fear causes us to lose control of our emotions. Fear may lead to panic and irrational behavior. Under the influence of fear, our reasoning processes are overwhelmed. Our sympathetic nervous system is involved. Reason, however, and a rational, realistic evaluation of the basis for fear, could lead to political and social steps to remove the cause of fear. For example, it has been established that terrorists are not crazy and poverty stricken, but intelligent members of the middle and upper classes, committing themselves to actions they believe will benefit their social peers. Finding the basis for changing such beliefs may be the approach to follow to reduce the basis of fear.

Loneliness affects young adults, and they find ways to cope with it. In a study by Rokach and Orzeck (2003), 818 subjects completed a 34-item questionnaire. A factor analysis identified six factors: Reflection and acceptance, Self-development and understanding, Social support network, Distancing and denial, Religion and faith, and Increased activity. The general population's responses were posed against the users of Ecstasy, a drug, and found that the drug users differed from the general population on several of the dimensions that were posed against loneliness.

Ecstasy users were lower on Reflection and acceptance and were somewhat lower on Self-development and understanding. On Distancing and denial, Ecstasy users differed from the non-drug users and the general population. Ecstasy users scored high on social support and Increased activity. A distressing and demeaning experience, loneliness depletes one's QOL. The study identifies ways of coping with it, with or without drugs. Social support stands as a major strategy: finding associates that cause one to cope. Reflection and acceptance provide the opportunity to gain self-understanding, a "joyous experience of self-discovery." Ecstasy users seek out others and avoid reflection on their situation. Non-Ecstasy users, on the other hand, do not seek out others and may be less likely to join organized groups. Establishing relationships with others is a pathway to remedying loneliness. The drug users scored higher than the other groups on Distancing and denial. The benefits of social support, also, are found in Religion and faith, providing an antidote to emptiness and meaninglessness. Increased activity, also, serves to combat loneliness. The study gives us insights, with or without Ecstasy, into the management of mood and loneliness, and thus it gives us keys to improving our QOL.

Love

Finding someone to love will enhance anyone's QOL. Love can alter one's identity, changing one's social position through attaching to another person. An identity change involves a change in social role, a change in status and power, hopefully increasing the satisfactions of one's QOL. Love involves two people; hence, it is a social as well as an individual status. Conversely, the loss of love involves a change in social role, status, and power, perhaps invoking sadness over the loss, with anxiety and heartache. Interacting in love between man and woman involves socially and culturally specified rituals. The symbolic engagement ring is followed upon marriage with the wedding ring, its presence acknowledged with festive parties and celebrations. The ritual marriage ceremony follows an established routine. There is legal recognition of the new relationship. Families of the couple become involved. The new status of husband and wife is socially, culturally, and legally recognized. Homosexual and lesbian relationships also represent love between two persons, attachments that provide security and identity.

C.S. Lewis, in his book *Four Loves*, discusses love in a broader context. Friendship is one basis of love: "that luminous, tranquil, rational world of relationships, freely chosen." Another is affection, involving both, according to Lewis, need-love and gift-love. Eros, erotic love, as represented above, includes sexual attraction. Lewis' fourth love is love of God, represented in a chapter headed "Charity," thereby acknowledging the social basis of love of God. Need-love is represented when one cannot get along without the other. Gift-love, on the other hand, Lewis characterizes as doing for the one you love. These two distinctions may be found in each of the four of Lewis' loves. It is an interesting concept, for love of various kinds pervades and contributes to the QOL.

Approaching love from a systems perspective, Sorokin (1950) developed a plan to improve the production of what he termed "love energy." He would increase the "heroes" of love, men like Homer and Dante, musical composers and religious leaders, like Buddha and St. Francis. Sorokin also proposed to increase the heroes of truth and beauty, which would increase love and "the field of goodness." Third, he proposed an increase in the production of love by the rank and file, however idealistic this may be. His exposition follows: "If the bulk of ordinary mortals would simply abstain from murdering other human beings; if they would cut in half their daily actions of hate and would double their daily good deeds, such a modest improvement in their moral conduct would enormously increase the output of love and decrease the output of hate, and thereby the general ethical and social level of humanity would be raised to a much higher level" (p. 67).

Sorokin also proposed an increase in the generation of love in groups and institutions, this, without the increase in animosity toward outside groups. Finally, he would increase the production of love by cultural systems and the total cultures, an even more idealistic proposal for an expansion of love.

Love can be characterized extensively. "God is love." "Love is patient and kind." "Love is learned." "One must love to be loved." "I love you." "One grows in love." "Love is an act of faith" (Buscaglia, 1972). "Love is now!" "There is no love where there is no will" (Gandhi). "Love cometh like sunshine after rain." "it is an ever-fixed mark, That looks on tempests, and is never shaken" (Shakespeare). "Love is a flame to set the will on fire" (John Masefield). "So sweet love seemed that April morn/ When first we kissed beside the thorn" (Robert Bridges). "Real love always creates" (Buscaglia, 1972). This could go on, but enough, enough.

Summary of Initiatives

Adapt and accommodate to negative emotions. They are part of life. Discipline is needed to control negative emotions. To achieve happiness, cultivate a tranquil state of mind, attending to others' happiness rather than seeking happiness directly for one's self.

Income to supply basic necessities is needed for happiness. Beyond that more money is not likely to bring more happiness.

To change attitudes:

Present information supporting the desired (new) attitude.
Use experts to persuade.
Instill beliefs consistent with the desired attitude.
Use role-playing for roles consistent with the desired attitude.
Employ reason and rationality to overcome fear.
Love another that you may serve another to enhance your QOL.

These are affective influences on our QOL. Our QOL is also influenced by cognitive, intellectual factors.

Chapter 5
Intellectual Autonomy

Or if it be virtue you love,
Why, virtues are the fruit of her (wisdom's) labors,
Since it is she who teaches temperance and patience,
Justice and fortitude.
–The Book of Wisdom, Ch. 8, verse 7, The Jerusalem Bible

Intelligence is quickness to apprehend as distinct from ability, which is capacity to act wisely on the thing apprehended.
–Dialogues of Alfred North Whitehead (1953), page 135

The whole art of teaching is only the art of awakening the natural curiosity of young minds for the purpose of satisfying it afterwards.
–Anatole France, The Crime of Sylvestre Bonnard, Part II, Chap. 4

Intellectual Autonomy. Being curious, broad-minded, creative, making mental progress, personal growth, social coherence. These are the products of a lifetime of learning, the institution of education, broadly conceived. Low intellectual autonomy relies upon others' judgments in decision-making, conforms to social pressures.

Proposition 5. The QOL may be enhanced by reducing illiteracy and low levels of education, and by expanding opportunities for formal and adult education, for personal growth in creativity, and for occasions to follow one's curiosity, thereby developing the inquiring mind.

Literacy

As a substitute for the concept of illiteracy, literacy was made the topic of statistics in a 1992 survey for the United States, followed by a second survey in 2003. The intervening 11-year-period showed an improvement in prose literacy for the lowest level of understanding prose. The two surveys determined prose literacy, document literacy, and mathematical literacy. For the United States, prose and document scores remained approximately constant between 1992 and 2003, but mathematical scores improved slightly. The lowest scores were among Hispanics and blacks.

A.L. Ferriss, *Approaches to Improving the Quality of Life*, Social Indicators Research   43
Series 42, DOI 10.1007/978-90-481-9148-2_5, © Springer Science+Business Media B.V. 2010

Based on a formula for estimating the lowest literacy level, the National Assessment of Adult Literacy has estimated the percent least literate by US county. This has pinpointed the literacy problem at its most elemental level, where steps may be taken to remedy the problem. South Carolina gave adult literacy classes to 80,000 and reduced its rate from 20 to 15% in 2003. Other states also have made progress.

Policymakers consider literacy essential to improve employability and citizenship. The more literate enjoy a more extensive QOL. The National Assessment of Adult Literacy (NAAL) may be accessed on the National Center for Education Statistics web site.

Education, Free Expression

One may achieve a productive and invigorating QOL when one has the freedom to think, speak, create, and express one's self. Such freedoms may be hampered by social conventions, such as prejudices and stereotypes that blindly restrict speech and activities. One may be hampered by political correctness, which may lead to untrue expressions. Individuals must discipline themselves against accepting such prejudices. They should employ conventional civility, and rationally assess people, events, and issues. There is a pathway to such rationality.

People may open doors to opportunities for self-development through formal or individual education. In the twenty-first century, acquiring academic degrees has become necessary in order to be recognized and has allowed the liberty for many creative endeavors. The extent of formal education required depends upon the profession and the skills, such as art or sculpture, acquired. Some studies show education positively associated with income and with happiness, but there are others that find income and occupation of greater significance to the QOL than education. However, being formally certified as competent gives an advantage. One's job performance then remains to seal one's competence.

Educating the Child

Improving the child's formal education involves massive interventions. Family life affects the child's scholarly standing, for children who watch TV 4 or 5 h daily score poorly on standardized tests, according to studies by the Educational Testing Service. Other limiting factors include absences from school, parents who do not read to offspring, and children living with only one parent. These conditions may be changed only through altering the treatment children receive from their parents. Education of parents in the proper care and nurturing of the child is required in order to prepare the child for best school performance.

The differential effect of father or mother upon the child's education has been reviewed for 30 countries by Marks (2008). He found that in most countries, the father's occupational status has a greater impact on student achievement than the mother's work situation. Educational status of parents, however, has the opposite effect – the mother's education carries more weight than the father's. When occupational status and educational status are combined, however, as one might expect, the influence is about equal in most countries. Marks attempted to classify countries according to their linguistic, economic, and cultural similarities, but was unable to identify any commonalities among them. The results, then, appear to be independent of socio-cultural factors in the 30 countries. Marks thinks that the influence of the mother is increasing.

Beginning in the 1980s, Taiwan expanded its higher education system. Since then, the educational differential between men and women has declined. A study by Lin and Yang (2009) traces the trend in educational inequality, showing the rapid decline in educational inequality of women and of men. They show that the labor force in some occupations is overly educated for the required tasks but acknowledge other benefits from education.

Flourishing

To flourish, according to Webster, is to grow luxuriantly, to thrive, to prosper, to reach a height of development or influence. One may have a flourishing QOL through freedom from the restrictions of negative emotions and freedom to develop intellectually. Cultivating interests and satisfying curiosity leads to pleasure of discovery and understanding. These are the keys to a flourishing and exciting existence. Although some leisure is required, these engagements can be attained regardless of level of income, marital or social status. (See Chapter 2 , Keyes on flourishing.)

Perhaps affective and intellectual autonomy are the true answers to achieving a desirable QOL. In *Experience and Education*, John Dewey said, "The only freedom that is of enduring importance is freedom of intelligence, that is to say, freedom of observation and judgment exercised in behalf of purposes that are intrinsically worthwhile."

Increasing the percentage of the population that is literate also involves promoting higher levels of formal and informal school and college education. For this one assumes that exposure to the vast arena of knowledge will enable intellectual independence and creativity in problem solving. Van Gundy (1981) has identified six principles for encouraging creativity, and his volume lists many procedures to help the teacher plan classroom activities to stimulate problem solving and creativity. The six principles include the following:

1. "Separate idea generation from evaluation," that is, when an idea is generated by an individual or group, do not immediately evaluate the efficacy of the idea in relation to the problem. Evaluation may come much later in the sequence of idea generation.

2. "Test assumptions." Once a creative idea has emerged from the thinking process, questions should be asked to explore the assumptions underlying the idea. The journalist's guidelines apply: ask what, why, when, who, where. Asking questions may lead to improved understanding of the problem and the creative idea for its solution.
3. "Avoid patterned thinking." We follow habit, in action, thought, and speech. Breaking habitual responses by consciously rejecting them may lead to fresh orientation, and more creative ideas.
4. "Create new perspectives." This involves examining the problem from a different viewpoint from the habitual, usual one. Turn it around. Look at it with another's eyes. This may lead to a new awareness of the problem and its creative solution.
5. "Minimize negative thinking." We tend to reject the unfamiliar, the new, until we have become more familiar with them. Critically rejecting a newly created idea gets us nowhere. Rather, the approach should begin by asking what is good about it, by identifying what we like about the new idea, and viewing it as "raw material" for action. Saying "no" will deny the chances of the new creative idea.
6. "Take prudent risks." To succeed with a new creative idea requires taking chances. The probability of success is not always 100%. New ideas and enterprises must be carried out with persistence and initiative that will ensure some degree of success. Risks are inherent in launching new thinking solutions. This must be acknowledged and the chances of failure minimized.

Van Gundy (2005), in his volume of activities, presents in detail the steps and processes for group leaders to follow in stimulating small groups to creative endeavors.

Creativity in Problem Solving

To teach creativity, the teacher must understand the creative process. The psychologist Eliot D. Hutchinson has outlined this process, emphasizing the role of *insight*. Insight, he says, is "the normal, the successful, the only sure way toward creative accomplishment" (Hutchinson, 1949, p. 16). He outlines four stages of the insight process. The first is the stage of preparation or orientation to the problem, involving assembling information on aspects of the problem. Then follows a stage of frustration during which no solution appears to the thinker who, perhaps, turns to other matters.

Next follows a period of insight, unanticipated and unpredictable, ideas arriving in a flash. Hutchinson gives many examples of insight by creative thinkers, scientists, poets, inventers, novelists, and many others. Insight may come when one is not consciously engaged with the problem, an observation Sigmund Freud attributed to the unconscious. Hutchinson believes insight comes under three conditions: "during or just after periods of rest and relaxation; in periods characterized by a slight mental abstraction or dissociation which in itself furnishes a momentary relaxation;

during periods of light physical activity, usually of a more or less repetitive and automatic character, which give relief from the insistent tensions involved" (p. 120). The teacher of creativity, then, must allow students these conditions in order to stimulate creativity.

What will be the student's reaction? The student will need time for creative ideas to germinate. When presented with a problem, the student will need skills to assemble the data or evidence required. The "frustration" phrase of the creative process will require additional time. How long before the insight dawns on the student? These and other hurdles may pose difficulties when such a study unit is entered into the curriculum.

Working with Conflict: Written by Dr. Margaret S. Herrman

Conflict surfaces when people in any type of relationship perceive independence and also perceive that their values, goals, interests, or actions are incompatible with or interfere with the values, goals, interests, or actions of others in the interaction (Herrman, 2005).

Conflicts typically exist long before anyone openly acknowledges a problem and asks for redress (Felsitner, Abel, & Sarat, 1980–1981). But, why delay? What are the options? Herrman (1994) describes several options, with avoidance being a favored response. (e.g., think how often you hear statements like: "If it's not broken, don't fix it." "Let's appoint a committee to study it." or "It's not THAT bad/important. It can wait." All indicate avoidance.) What little we know tells us that, depending on the type of conflict, a minimum of 75% of the time, avoidance is the first response, and sometimes the only response to a conflict.

Avoidance is not always bad. We know from social psychology that avoidance makes perfect sense when an interaction is not highly valued and the other person involved can be replaced easily. If the interaction is fleeting and involves a stranger, avoidance is a great response. But, on any given day how many interactions involve strangers who are easily replaced? For most interactions, those that involve ongoing relationships and especially those involving people who are near and dear, avoid avoidance. Why? Avoidance submerges a conflict, leaving all the sources of friction in place and raw. By not complaining about a problem, the offender continues to operate in the dark with no opportunity to address the concern. All the while the offense continues to rankle, sometimes resulting in "unrealistic conflicts" (see Coser, 1956, 1961) and polarization. Both contribute to future conflicts that are harder to solve and more destructive than the original problem.

Once the limitations of avoidance are clear, you begin to look at strategies for confronting a conflict. Simply, they reduce to either: "I try to win and you lose." or "I lose, and you win." or "We both give something up." or "We take time to talk and listen to discern the nature of the problem, our individual and collective resources, and possible solutions."

Our individualistic culture (Augsburger, 1992) reinforces a win/lose, zero-sum mind-set. The mind-set helps to explain avoidance since we have less than a 50/50 chance of winning, especially if you factor in the third option, compromise. The fourth strategy of talking, listening, and collaborating on a solution that meets everyone's needs flies in the face of a culture that values quick fixes, a John Wayne or Clint Eastwood minimalist communicator style, and a winner take all metaphor. So, how do you talk and listen with the intent of "do no harm?"

Suggestions for Confronting Positively

There are many steps that can help. This is only a beginning.

1. Not all conflicts call for "a solution" or closure, indeed very few do. Issues and ideas we hold dear never go away. They might be solved for the moment, but the word (re)solved is more accurate. Important issues surface repeatedly. They morph as we find new ways of working with others, but the issues remain (e.g., issues related to sex and money in a marriage).
2. Conflict is ubiquitous, a component of any sustained interaction, but not unidimensional. Different roots hold different implications for outcomes. The literature describes numerous sources of conflict, including conflicts over values, relations, structures, interests, and data (Felsitner et al., 1980–1981). Under this nomenclature, structural conflicts are generally easier to solve than either relational or values conflicts which resonate deeply with someone's sense of self. So, first think about the source of a conflict, and only then project a reasonable outcome. Expect data conflicts to be resolved, but values and even relational conflicts might call for dialogue and the creation of mutual respect for diverse ways of thinking and interacting. Outcomes might bring temporary closure or respect for differing views or understanding. All are valuable, just very different.
3. Prepare for a confrontation.

    – Make a cognitive shift from having a debate to being in dialogue, to having a fruitful conversation with someone you value. The shift requires doing your homework. Gather the information you might need to inform the other person. If data needs to be collected (say sales receipts or comparable quotes), collect it, and create some way of easily displaying the data (the goal is to enhance understanding of a point of view, not overwhelm or dazzle).
    – Reflect on how and what you are feeling. Explore why you feel what you do. Saying "I statements" to yourself helps (you might later use the same statements when discussing the problem with the other person). Here you mull over something like: "I get angry, when you ... ... (a specific act or circumstance). I want you to ... ... (your preferred change)."
    – Another useful technique involves triangulation. Triangulation means you are talking to a third person about the situation. Triangulation is a form of grapevine if there is no agreement about confidentiality and if you only talk to the third person and not the person directly involved (a bad move). But, if you ask a third person to maintain your confidence (and they do), and your intent

is to rehearse or just "spit it out," the technique helps you explore feelings and gives you valuable feedback from someone not directly involved.

4. Whether trying to resolve a conflict or reach mutual understanding, begin by creating an environment for safe, unrushed conversation that supports respectful talking and listening. Tell the other person you need to work on a conflict together, but only after you agree on procedures or how and when you can discuss the situation. Seek support from the other person so you all allocate time to talk (and possibly to talk more than once) and a place where you have privacy (unless there is a potential for violence in the interaction – that calls for a whole different set of circumstances). A good way to initiate a preliminary conversation is to express your commitment to the relationship, your desire to understand, and your hope that change will support the relationship.

5. Once you arrive at the time and place for confronting a problem, be prepared to talk and even more to listen. Be curious. Be compassionate. Be open. Slow down (your breathing, your thinking, your heart rate); try not to rush or over talk the other person. You will learn a lot from what the other person has to say, and also from hearing yourself explain what is going on. Do not be surprised if you learn that what you want and need is not so at odds with the wants and needs of the other person.

6. Create a mutual feeling that it is safe to talk. Mediators are trained to create rapport that supports talking, listening, and a perception that the other person hears what you are saying.

7. Do not assume you know or interpret what the other person is saying correctly. If you are normal, you are probably doing just the opposite. Less than 10% of all communication is accurate. So, ask questions for clarification and out of heartfelt curiosity.

8. Finally, if the goal is to support change after the discussion, think about eight ways of successful action plans. In your conversation, it would be great if you can cover all eight:

   – What is the problem, the issue, or concern?
   – Why are these problems, issues, or concerns important to you? How do they impact the other person?
   – What needs to be done, what needs to change (an attitude, actions, procedures, the use of specific words or gestures in conversations, arrangement of the furniture, etc.)?
   – Where will these changes take place?
   – When will the changes take place – what are the priorities and time line?
   – Who is responsible for completing each change?
   – What resources do people need to be successful?
   – When do we come back and evaluate/assess progress and update the game plan? (End of Margaret Herrman's discussion.)

Remember that conflict is a natural part of all human interaction. Conflict, per se, is neither good nor bad. It just is. In fact, social interactions become stale, rigid, and dysfunctional in the absence of conflict. What is truly important is how someone reacts to a conflict. There are simple choices and actions that help insure successful outcomes for supporting everyone in a social interaction. Enjoy your options. Use them often (Van Gundy, 1981).

Conclusion

In summary, intellectual autonomy requires literacy, gained through formal education and individual and child and adult education. Free intellectual development contributes to a flourishing QOL. In solving problems, creativity, and tested procedures for conflict resolution, as Herman has outlined, lay out a clear track to follow. Problems always will be with us. It is how we manage them that will contribute to a better QOL.

Chapter 6
Harmony

This royal throne of kings, this scepter'd isle,
This earth of majesty, this seat of Mars,
This other Eden, demi-paradise,
This fortress built by Nature for herself
Against infection and the hand of war,
This happy breed of men, this little world,
This precious stone set in the silver sea,
Which serves it in the office of a wall
Or as a moat defensive to a house,
Against the envy of less happier lands,
This blessed plot, this earth, this realm, this England...
            –William Shakespeare, King Richard III, Act II, Sc. 1.

Come live with me, and be my love;
And we will all the pleasures prove
That hills and valleys, dales and fields,
Woods or sleepy mountains yields.
            –Christopher Marlowe, The Passionate Shepherd to His Love

How often we forget all time, when lone,
Admiring Nature's universal throne,
Her woods, her wilds, her waters, the intense
Reply of hers to our intelligence.
            –George Noel Gordon, Lord Byron, The Island, Canto II, Stanza 16

Harmony. A non-toxic environment, enjoying the world of beauty, the feeling of a unity of nature, sustaining environmental mastery. Control of external activities that affect well-being. Low harmony results from inability to change or improve the surrounding context, lack of sense of control over external world.

Proposition 6. The QOL may be enhanced by reducing and eliminating environmental toxins and other impediments to a harmonious Nature, by working for a sustainable environment, and by encouraging the work of environmental groups, such as the Sierra Club and similar organizations.

A.L. Ferriss, *Approaches to Improving the Quality of Life*, Social Indicators Research Series 42, DOI 10.1007/978-90-481-9148-2_6, © Springer Science+Business Media B.V. 2010

Toxins

Environmental toxins in land, air, and water adversely affect QOL by increasing morbidity and mortality. Various studies have shown air pollution to result in lung damage in children, lung cancer, fetal deaths, and infant mortality, including sudden death syndrome, respiratory illness, and death from respiratory infections, cardiovascular disease, skin problems, ulcers, and liver and kidney damage, premature deaths, and asthma (Lauer & Lauer, 2006).

Environmental pollution results from industrial manufacturing processes, automobile exhausts, pesticides and herbicides employed in agricultural production, garbage disposal, and other sources. The Council on Environmental Quality (United States) has identified the major chemical and other pollutants, which include "total suspended particulates, sulfur dioxide, carbon monoxide, petrochemical oxidants, nitrogen dioxide, and hydrocarbons." Three of these (carbon monoxide, nitrogen oxide, and hydrocarbons) are attributed to automobile exhaust. The Council on Environmental Quality suggests the following controls of these emissions, as reported by Lauer and Lauer (2006, pp. 438–439).

For control of carbon monoxide: "Automobile engine modifications (including tuning, exhaust gas recirculation, design of combustion chamber, control of automobile exhaust gases (catalytic or thermal devices), improved design, operation and maintenance of stationary furnaces (use of finely dispersed fuels, proper mixing with air, high combustion temperature)."

For control of nitrogen oxide: "Catalytic control of automobile exhaust gases, modification of automobile engines to reduce combustion temperatures, scrubbing flue gases with caustic substances or urea."

For control of hydrocarbons: "Automobile engine modifications (proper tuning, crankcase ventilation, exhaust gas recirculation, redesign of combustion chamber); control of automobile exhaust gases (catalytic or thermal devices); improved design, operation and maintenance of stationary furnaces (use of finely dispersed fuels, proper mixing with air, high combustion temperature); improved control procedures in processing and handling petroleum compounds." (Lauer & Lauer, 2006, quoting the Council on Environmental Quality).

Most of the preceding involves technical manufacturers' actions. As consumers, we could promote purchase of vehicles that include these improvements.

Land Pollution

According to Lauer and Lauer (2006, pp. 440–462), other sources of environmental polluting include land pollution by pesticides, herbicides, chemical wastes, etc., water pollution, global warming, noise pollution, deterioration of the beauty of the environment, and others.

Factors contributing to environmental pollution include population growth that exceeds the carrying capacity of the environment and industrial basis of the economy. Newspaper accounts say that about 1.4 billion people worldwide lack a source of safe drinking water. About half that number lives without proper sanitation. They estimate that contaminated drinking water causes death to an estimated five million children annually.

Toxic environments are identified by geographic clusters of mortality due to cancer or other causes. Chemists analyze the soil to discover the cause. For example, Gorahm, a large silver manufacturer of Providence, RI, employed electroplating and metalwork that contaminated the soil. Childhood leukemia affected children in Woburn, MA, as described in *No Safe Place* by Phil Brown and Edwin Mikelsen. Blue soil was discovered recently at Tiverton, RI, caused by contamination with arsenic, a deadly poison, and other chemicals from a manufactured gas plant. The local government declared that no digging in the soil would be allowed. Some 120 homes were affected in the Bay Street Neighborhood.

Citizens conduct surveys of their neighborhood to identify prevalence of disease conditions, extent of contaminated drinking water, and other factors that may indicate a nearby source of contamination. Often they engage environmental agencies of the state to assist. Social scientists are called in to assess the ecological aspects, with chemists and other disciplines being involved.

Water

In South America and Africa, corporations have developed water projects that have not benefited poor people. Fees are charged for connecting to water-supply sources. Corporations demand a profit from their development.

In some underdeveloped areas, especially in Africa, the contaminated water supply retards individual development and, as a consequence, socioeconomic development of the region. Tests show the water is contaminated with pathogens that cause diseases, such as diarrhea, dysentery, typhoid, and cholera. The consequence is a depleted QOL. In the Niger-Delta River region of Nigeria, the deficiency in water supply amounts to 68% of the demand, according to a study by Nkwocha (2009). The region has been neglected by government policies for generations, based upon ethnic disparities and political, economic, and social insecurities.

Global Warming

Looking to the future, say 2050 and beyond, global warming will impact farming practices and production. In the warmer regions, in America from the southern states in the United States to the south of Brazil, carbon emissions will likely reduce agricultural crop yields. Similarly, African countries and southern Asia will suffer reductions. The loss may be lessened by change to crops more tolerant of heat. On the other hand, the northern sectors where agriculture production has been minor will increase in productivity. Corn production is likely to decline. Rice production will decline in regions subject to excessive flooding. These changes in supply of food will take place in a world of increasing demand through population increases. Solutions to these crop problems lie in reducing carbon emissions, adjusting agricultural production to avoid loss of food supply, and moving toward lower rates of population increase. To avoid worldwide reduction in the QOL, adjustments will be needed both in food production and demographic growth.

These observations and predictions were reinforced in a US Department of Agriculture commission report on US Climate Change Science Program. Some 38 scientists examined more than 1,000 scientific papers on the impact of carbon dioxide emissions from burning fossil fuels. The consequence is currently being seen in more frequent forest fires, increased drought, and change in seasonal weather patterns. The report emphasized that these consequences are not 25 or 50 years in the future. They are now. For example, in Minqin County, China, a water reservoir for irrigation has dried up and become a desert. A rapidly warming climate has brought about the loss of permafrost affecting the Alaskan village of Shishmaref, causing houses to topple and the villagers to move to the mainland. In 2003, a heat wave in Europe caused the death of an estimated 35,000 people. Floods in 1998 affected 240 million Chinese, but in early 2009, drought took away proper drinking water of 4,400,000 Chinese. The government allocated $12 billion to help wheat production in north China.

The worldwide annual death toll from climate change is estimated at 150,000, according to the World Health Organization. The impact of climate change on the QOL requires adjustments in daily routines and attention to housing, outdoor exposure, management of livestock, reduction of emissions, and related measures. Reduction in emissions of carbon dioxide today has become urgent in order to preserve our current QOL and to leave a legacy of a sustainable climate to future generations.

The ethical principal involved here is that our behavior benefiting ourselves should not result in harm to others (Broome, 2008). By "others" is meant future generations who must live (or die) as consequence of the toxic emissions today. By living less lavishly today, eating less meat, traveling less, using less energy, and so forth, we improve the chances that future QOL will be sustainable. Economists have envisioned that reducing emissions of toxins today would benefit the future far greater than the cost to us today (a cost–benefit analysis). It involves sacrificing today in order to benefit tomorrow. Strong policies are needed now to control climate change.

Meat

The Worldwatch Institute in its *State of the World* reported that one-fifth of greenhouse gases emit from livestock. Some 37% of methane comes from effluvia of livestock. They release 65% of the carbon dioxide that rises to the sky. Altogether, animal agriculture releases 300 l of methane daily. It rises into the stratosphere to add to the chemical cover that causes our global warming. The United Nations reports that over half the world's arable land supports animals that we, in turn, eat. This includes cattle, sheep, poultry, pigs, and other animals. We cut down forests to clear land to grow soybeans, grains, and hay to feed the animals that we eat. On average in the United States, we consume 112 pounds of red meat and 72.2 pounds of poultry annually. Meat is not the healthiest food. It provides fat and protein, neither of which we require in abundance. Vegetables, grains, and fruits are better sources of proteins, fiber, antioxidants, and other nutrients. Our environment, our health, and our QOL would benefit if we abandoned meat and instead ate primarily vegetables and fruits.

Other Energy Sources

The environment responds to pollution from power-generating plants, such as coal burning electric plants, and nuclear plants. To reduce such pollution, other sources of energy are required.

One such source is ocean waves, the motion of which may be captured in turbines that generate electricity. Point absorbers, overlapping devices, attenuators, and oscillating water columns are various technologies that can be applied to turn wave power into electricity. However, operating and maintenance costs are estimated at 40% of production and the cost of a kilowatt-hour is estimated at 9 cents compared with 4–7 cents for wind power and 6–8 cents for new coal-fired power plants. Experimental developments, however, may change these estimates.

About 20% of US electrical power is generated by 140 nuclear power plants. These plants emit few emissions that contribute to global warming. Safety is a problem; since 1979, some 35 reactors have been shut down to restore a minimum level of safety. Reactors produce radioactive nuclear waste that must be stored in an isolated environment. The United States currently stores nuclear waste in casks encased in concrete and open, unfortunately, to terrorist attack. Yucca Mountain, Nevada, has been proposed as a safe location for storage. Enriched uranium goes into the nuclear power plants as fuel. It must be enriched by an enrichment plant.

To improve the safety of the power plants, the reactors can be constructed better than the present ones. The government can maintain greater oversight to the operation, and protection against attack can be improved. In addition, the nuclear waste problem must be addressed. Altogether, the prospect is promising that nuclear power can contribute to meeting the demand for electricity and help reduce emissions that cause global warming (Gronlund, 2008).

Electricity

Reducing environmental toxins will give us a cleaner environment. The generation of electricity by wind will provide a reliable and sustainable source of energy. The technology has been improved to the extent that since 1998, when wind generated approximately 2,000 MW of electricity, more than 12,000 MW were produced in 2006 (Dyette, 2006). Authorities have identified two possible advances in this technology: turbines placed in offshore wind would be more effective than land-based turbines, but would require advances in construction of stable platform foundations and transmission technologies. Land-based turbines would produce more were they built higher in order to take advantage of upper air speeds. Current wind production provides electricity for 2.5 million homes. The future will see this source of energy expand (Dyette, 2006).

The Union of Concerned Scientists, in its *Earthwise* newsletter (Summer, 2009), recommends that one-fourth of electricity be generated from renewable sources by 2025. The organization estimates this will create 297,000 jobs in the United States and save the public $64.3 billion by the target date. It also recommends that polluters be required to pay for their emissions that cause global warming.

A Five-Step Plan

James Hansen (2007) has outlined a five-step plan for meeting the global environmental crisis. He is the director of NASA's Goddard Institute for Space Studies. First, he would stop building coal-fired power plants until the technology is developed to filter carbon emissions from the process.

Second, he turns to economics, and would put a price on emissions, thereby increasing costs to users with the hope of reducing demand for such products.

Third, Hansen would establish energy-efficient standards, which would guide engineers and architects to reduce energy requirements of structures. Architects have said they can reduce energy requirements of buildings by 50%.

The fourth recommendation concerns ice-sheet stability; the topic is significant because the collapse of ice sheets would cause the oceans to rise 16–19 ft, bringing calamity to coastal cities. Hansen would ask the National Academy of Sciences to study the problem in order to find an intelligent solution.

Finally, Hansen would reform communication practices that involve the scientific community, the public, and the political process. He feels that scientific information is not being used by policy-makers due, in part, to uninformed political appointees who occupy critical public offices. He feels that the global warming problem is not readily resolved because of special interests that influence public policy to the detriment of intelligent action to reduce the causes of global warming (Hansen, 2007).

The University of Colorado, Denver School of Public Affairs has a Presidential Action Climate Project. Its recommendations may be found on www.climateactionproject.com. Its recommendations ask that federal subsidies be reformed to discourage the use of fossil fuels and encourage renewable energy, especially including wind and solar power. It also recommends combining the US Small Business Administration with the Department of Energy offices in order to facilitate technology innovations relative to energy. Energy costs are important in its recommendations.

The key to several of these problems lies in transforming environmental forces into energy. Energy from Middle Eastern oil drains fiscal resources, and the use of oil results in carbon dioxide in the atmosphere. A solution to both of these problems lies in transforming environmental forces into energy.

Electricity may be generated by tapping into thermal vents under the sea at various points, one being Hawaii. Most available, also, is the force of wind. Wind farms generate electricity, especially bordering seacoast lines. Another approach is the manufacture of ethanol for fuel. It may be processed not only from corn and other grains but also from algae, palm trees, sugar, and other such products. Solar energy may be trapped for energy of buildings. Such installations in Hawaii government buildings are said to eliminate the demand for 130,000 barrels of oil a year. Tapping geothermal energy from hot pockets below volcanoes provides another possibility.

The target for Hawaii aims at producing 70% of its energy from renewable sources by 2030. Other states with different environmental resources could aim for similar reduction in the use of oil.

Former vice president Al Gore heads an Alliance for Climate Protection. He advocates removing carbon-based energy sources by obtaining energy from solar panels, windmills, nuclear energy, natural gas, clean coal, and dams to harness waterpower. Over a 30-year period, the transition would cost an estimated 1.5 trillion to 3 trillion dollars. A bipartisan organization, Securing America's Future Energy, maintains that fossil fuels can be eliminated over a 10-year-period. Both groups seek to solve the global warming problem. It, like dirty drinking water, deters a flourishing QOL.

The Israeli government has adopted a plan to reduce emissions from automobiles. It has asked automakers to produce electric vehicles. By 2011, the transition is expected to begin. It will be completed by 2020, at which time the country will no longer depend upon gasoline. The roads will be spotted with electric recharging stations.

Urban Renewal

Urban environments vary in density. Previous studies have suggested that, as population density increases, there is a decline in perceived QOL and living conditions. New studies, however, employing numerous scales of various aspects of living, have not substantiated this conclusion. Instead, a study of Auckland, New Zealand, and two cities in northern Italy found that residents rated most living conditions favorably in medium-density neighborhoods. The studies included a variety of aspects of living, which, taken together, contribute to the QOL. The authors (Walton et al., 2008) conclude that population density has no significant effect upon most aspects of living conditions.

Humans Adapt

Cultural conditioning undoubtedly has an effect, as does tradition, on the manifest capacity of humans to adjust to adverse conditions of living. A different conclusion is made by a study of a sample of 2065 Swedes (Cramer et al., 2004). Low, negative correlations were found with population density and subjective well-being and global QOL ($r = -0.12$ and -0.15). Education and income were held constant. This gives some support, though weak, with the original conclusion of the adverse influence of population density. The topic remains to be explored further.

In an urban environment, urban planners may alter conditions of living to improve housing, superstructure of streets and buildings, and so forth. A study of urban renewal in Hong Kong has demonstrated that renewal improves the QOL of residents. The study found that the resident with a higher level of education was less affected by renewal than were less-educated residents. It found that the resident's subjective QOL during urban renewal was not negatively influenced by his perception of the quality of the environment. Thus, urban renewal positively impacts QOL and is a sure means of improving residents' subjective well-being (Cheung & Leung, 2008).

Summary of Actions Needed

Technology

Most actions to improve the environment require technological developments. We call upon science to devise reductions in emissions from machines and to improve sources of energy. Energy providers, also, must initiate change for the benefit of economic and social conditions.

The technological changes needed are as follows:
Generate electricity from wind, water, and geothermal sources.
Stop building coal-fired power plants.
Seek a solution to ice-sheet instability.
Modify automobile engines to reduce emissions of pollutants.
Social and economic efforts that will contribute include the following:
Slow population growth, zero growth being the goal.
In response to global warning, adjust agricultural production in warmer and formerly cold geographic regions.
Improve architectural features of buildings so as to conserve energy.
Increase the price of electricity in order to reduce demand.
Scientists and others should improve communication to policy-makers of scientific results concerning environmental pollution.
Urbanites may improve QOL through renewing their environment.

Lower fertility in high-fertility regions will slow population growth and reduce energy demand.

Turning from meat to vegetables and fruit will help reduce environmental pollution and help reduce global warming.

For future generations to enjoy a flourishing QOL, many of these strategies are essential.

Chapter 7
Conservatism

It is preoccupation with possession, more than anything else,
that prevents men from living freely and nobly.
— Bertrand Russell, Principles of Social Reconstruction.

Happy the man and happy he alone,
He, who can call today his own:
He who, secure within, can say,
Tomorrow do thy worst, for I have lived today.
— Horace, bk .iii, ode xxix, trans. by John Dryden.

In the multitude of counselors there is safety.
—Proverbs 11:14

Conservatism. Maintaining social order, self-discipline, family security, safety, security obtained through work and productive activity results in social integration.

Proposition 7. The QOL may be enhanced by reducing or eliminating the causes for public disorder, riots, and terrorism, and by improving family and neighborhood security, strengthening individual self-discipline and security through work and other productive activity.

Whatever disturbs the peace and tranquility of the society comes under the domain of *conservatism*. This covers a wide territory. Under other topics, we have discussed several disturbing situations: riots and hate groups under *egalitarian commitment*, disturbances of happiness under *affective autonomy*, threats of violence that challenge *survival*, and others. Still, other topics remain. On the job discord may lead to unhappiness at home. Most anyone who walks down an urban street may fall victim to violence, and there are terrorism and other menaces that "flesh is heir to." We cannot address them all, but we can identify a few and set forth precautionary rules for guidance in the interest of a better QOL.

Violence

Violence occurs against women in the form of rape, against Jews, historically, and against African-Americans as a part of an age-old struggle for their human rights. Natives harbor violence against the new immigrant, the stranger. In the United

States, residents target aggression against Hispanics. For the present, Protestants and Catholics in Northern Ireland have quieted their traditional animosity. In other regions, religious groups stand against one another. Muslims terrorize against Western culture and against other religious thinking. Humankind violates human rights and disrupts the QOL through violence because of religion, ethnicity, gender, and other differences.

Baumbaugh-Smith, Gross, Wollman, and Yoder (2008) have developed a National Index of Violence and Harm that shows a decided decline in interpersonal violence in the United States between 1995 and 2003. Observers have found deaths from substance abuse increasing, but others declining: homicide, sexual offenses, battery, robbery, reckless behavior, and self-injury/suicide. He and associates found social negligence increasing. In the index, they included the high school dropout rate, which increased slightly. Other measures showing an increase were lack of health insurance, hunger (some 12.5 million households experiencing food shortage), and homelessness. People ages 15–29 years commit crimes at higher rates than others, according to US arrest rates. Thus, violence rates are influenced by the changing age distribution.

Conflict

Karl Marx set forth a theory of conflict generated by the disparate interests of workers and the owners of the means of production. Capitalism, he said, created conditions that lead to crime and violence. He proposed as a solution that workers own the means of production. Class conflict would be eliminated. Marx's theory has been expanded into a conflict theory and under-girds much sociological research today. For example, income inequality has been found to lead to higher homicide rates. Limited opportunities for economic and political progress may lead to riots that disturb the peace. Discouraged immigrants, even second and third generation immigrants, in some European countries, have felt isolated from mainstream society and have rioted.

Conflict, according to Georg Simmel, a German sociologist, may integrate people into groups and bring about needed social change, perhaps benefiting the QOL. Conservatives favor security and peace to conflict and confrontation. They may think differently when their security is threatened.

Poverty

The causes of riots in various countries may differ, depending upon the nature of the grievance, but income inequality lies at the heart of many. In 1981, the world had 1.5 billion people living in extreme poverty, more than half of them in east Asia and the Asian Pacific. (The various definitions of poverty are discussed in Chapter 3,

Mastery, q.v.) Since then, the global economy has expanded, spreading wealth to many less fortunate lands. By 2001, those in extreme poverty had shrunk to 1.1 billion, the largest number, 431 million living in south Asia. Sub-Saharan Africa has experienced an increase in extreme poverty, from 164 million in 1981 to 313 million in 2001. Extreme poverty in east Asia and the Pacific, meanwhile, with a growing population, has declined from 796 million in 1981 to 271 million in 2001. South Asia and sub-Saharan Africa remain the most deprived, hungry sectors. To reduce income inequality, lower poverty, and improve the QOL, the world strategy has been to develop the country economically, as Moss (1999) has written, to create wealth to improve living conditions. To impact poverty, countries must distribute a larger share of income to those in direst need, through jobs, education, health, and other benefits.

Disease, isolation, illiteracy, hunger, and other deprivations beset poverty-stricken areas. Countries of the west, and others that enjoy a higher QOL, have turned their attention to finding a solution to the problem of extreme poverty. The theory holds that the production of wealth in the form of goods and services lies at the basis of economic prosperity. Economic development is generated by investment of international corporations in poorer nations. Studies have not been unanimous in showing long-term benefits to these countries, but with recent changes in the global economy, foreign investments in poorer nations are showing long-term as well as short-term benefits.

A new measure, PPP – purchasing power parity – enables comparisons across nations. In 2002, the US value of PPP was $36,111 per capita, when about 13% of the population was in poverty, according to the US Census definition. European nations show a PPP value of $16,150 per capita. South central Asian nations show PPP per capita value of $2,370, while eastern African nations rank lowest with a per capita PPP of $800, and middle African nations $1,000 per capita. These figures express the extent of the poverty problem for sub-Saharan Africa, with 693 million people, and Asia, except China, with 2,485 million. With these numbers, the popular notion that 50% of the world's population lives in poverty seems reasonable.

Pollard and Lee (2003) reviewed recent studies of child well-being and found orientations in five domains: physical, psychological, cognitive, social, and economic. Only the psychological domain identified negative deficit indicators involving emotions, mental health, or illness. Intellectual or school-related factors identified the cognitive domain. A measure of child well-being should employ multiple dimensions, according to the study. This conclusion arose because some 80% of the studies examined employed only one domain to measure child well-being. They concluded that both subjective and objective factors should be employed to measure a child's performance. Child strengths as well as deficits should be examined in developing an adequate measure of well-being.

Two scholars, Delamonica and Minujin (2007), have developed a more refined method of defining poverty of children. Following E. S. Gordon and associates, they used seven factors of deprivation of children to estimate the number in developing countries. The number with one or more poverty indicators in the five UN regions sums to 1,028,805 children living in 46 developing countries. The items of deprivation were identified by E.S. Gordon and associates in their book, *The Distribution of Child Poverty in the Developing World* (Policy Press, Bristol University), as follows:

(1) Severe nutrition deprivation;
(2) Severe water deprivation;
(3) Severe deprivation of sanitation facilities;
(4) Severe health deprivation;
(5) Severe shelter deprivation;
(6) Severe education deprivation;
(7) Severe information deprivation.

Each of these deprivations is specifically defined. For our interests in finding pathways to improve the QOL, the seven deprivations outline the type of living conditions we must address in order to bring the poorest in the world to a better QOL.

Muhammad Yunus was awarded the Nobel Peace Prize in 2006 for starting the Grameen Bank in Bangladesh in 1976. It furnished small loans to poor individuals with no collateral for the support of small enterprises. Repayment was overseen by local committees, largely women, with 98% returns. Yunus did not invent the program, which the Ford Foundation sponsored in Asia some years earlier with successful results. The microfinance idea has been active also in Kenya, where some 17,000 borrowers have benefited from the loans. The microcredit system has been urged as a program for the World Bank. It holds promise for alleviating poverty at its grass-roots level, and improving the QOL of the most impoverished. (See Chapter 3 on Small Business Loans.)

Identity Theft

A serious crime, identity theft occurs when someone uses another's good name and credit record, social security number, bank account, and other identities and profits therefrom without the owner's knowledge. Identity theft can drastically affect one's peace and QOL. When the crime is eventually discovered, the victim may spend thousands of dollars and months or years cleaning up the mess.

Criminals may acquire identity information by stealing mail or discarded documents. They may rummage through trash. They may pose as an employer, landlord, or other person having a legal right to the information. They may steal credit card numbers and order merchandize with delivery by mail. They may steal a purse or wallet. They may use a change of address form to redirect mail to an address available to them. They may steal the information from a home. Using pretexting by phone, they may pose as legitimate companies with rights to the information.

Using the information for illegal gain may follow various paths. By changing the address of a credit card, it may be used for sometime without the victim's knowledge, the statements coming to an address other than the legitimate owner's. Identity thieves may open a new credit card in another's name, then leave the bills unpaid, thereby damaging the person's credit record. They may establish a phone or wireless service in someone else's name. They may counterfeit checks or debit cards in another's name, authorize transfers and drain the bank account. They may buy a car by taking out an auto loan in someone else's name. They have been known to get a drivers license with their picture using someone else's name. During an arrest, they may give another's name and identity to police and not show up for a court date, resulting in a warrant for arrest issued in the innocent person's name.

If one's identity is stolen, one should alert credit bureaus to the theft and close accounts that have been compromised or that were opened fraudulently. One should file a complaint with the proper governmental authority, the Federal Trade Commission. One should file an identity theft report, setting forth the details of the theft as they are known (Federal Trade Commission, 2009).

Criminal Justice System

The system of police, courts, attorneys, corrections, etc., has the objective of enforcing laws and maintaining order. Without such a system, anarchy and disorder would likely prevail, causing fear and destroying the QOL. Each community maintains its criminal justice system, creating variation in the extent to which laws are enforced and order maintained. Crime rates, both by type of crime and the magnitude of rates, vary by region in the United States. For example, violent crime is more prevalent in the south (542.6/100,000 population) and in the northeast less prevalent (393.6/100,000). The District of Columbia has the highest rate of violent crime and North Dakota the lowest. Other forms of crime, also, vary by state and region: murder and manslaughter, rape, robbery, aggravated assault, property crime, robbery, larceny/theft, and motor vehicle theft. These are types of crime tracked by the Uniform Crime Reporting System of the US Department of Justice.

Crime also is reckoned by the US National Crime Victimization Survey, a household interview, which produces statistics that are greater than those reported to the police for the Uniform Crime Report. In 2005, 23.4 million victimizations were reported for persons 12 years and older. There were 21.2 violent crimes per 1,000 population. Attacks with a weapon or other object that caused serious injury affected 4.3/1,000, while simple assault was more frequent (13.5/1,000). Property crimes were the most frequently reported, 154/1,000. The survey shows that violent crimes have declined in recent years, owing partly to the decline in the number of persons of ages committing most offences.

A study of victimization in Prince George, British Columbia, Canada, concluded that crime issues had little impact upon happiness, QOL, or life satisfaction. The study combined three measures: satisfaction with friendships, financial security, and health, satisfaction with personal and family safety, and beliefs about crime increase. Taken together, these satisfaction measures explained only 5% of the variance in a happiness measure. It could also explain 7% of the life satisfaction score, and 9% of the satisfaction with the QOL. However, when a broader measure of life circumstances was posed against the crime measure, the investigators found little to blame on victimization. Other life circumstances were more important to the people's QOL than concern about crime (Michalos & Zumbo, 2000).

Policing services of Prince George, B.C., were assessed by a sample of 698 residents in May of 2001 (Michalos, 2003). Overall, citizens favorably evaluated the Prince George police services. In addition to the assessment, the effect of policing services on the quality of life was measured in five different ways. Some 68% of respondents believed the local police were doing a good job and only 2% thought they were doing a "very poor job." The sample of citizens most favorably appreciated the police work aimed at preventing crime. For example, people were instructed to conceal items left in automobiles, to reduce theft. Prince George community was surveyed in 1971, as reported above (Michalos & Zumbo, 2000). Fewer people in the 2001 survey than in 1971 thought crime was increasing, and criminal justice statistics in fact show crime was not increasing. Respondents listed speeding and careless driving as two of the biggest problems, but these infractions were not high on the list of the police. They think highly of the work the police do to prevent crime. The survey measured QOL with five different indicators. Only satisfaction with police services was significantly associated with three of the QOL indicators. Satisfaction with policing services did not rank high in relation to happiness and life satisfaction. Happiness and life satisfaction, rather, were related to five of six other predictors: "your living partner," "your friendships," "your health," "your self esteem," "your job." These same domains were significantly related to QOL, with local policing services, also, related. Sixty-two percent of the variance in QOL was explained by these variables. Seventy-six percent of the variance in subjective well-being was found to be common with nine predictors, including policing services.

These results show policing services to make a positive contribution to QOL, although other, more intimate factors, also figure in people's evaluations. Protection from crime and other such sources of insecurity loom large in people's QOL.

People break the law for many reasons. The need for money causes many crimes. There are fraud and other white-collar crimes, largely for money. There are gangs of young men organized to distribute unlawful drugs. Persons of a different culture from the predominant US culture may commit acts that are not a crime in their culture but are defined as a crime in the United States. An example, committed by persons of Middle Eastern culture, is murder of a female family member to uphold family honor. Juveniles sometimes commit delinquencies for the thrill of it. The cause of crime is endless. Whatever the cause, crime impacts the QOL.

Victims of crime are affected by fear, alienation, economic loss, injury, and other ills. Crime depletes the QOL. The government has the responsibility of crime control and maintaining order. To achieve a better QOL, each domain herein presented advocates law abiding behavior. Abiding by the tenets of a free market society, cultivating attitudes and beliefs supportive of the community, becoming creative in intellectual or artistic pursuits, acting on behalf of a clean and toxin-free environment, avoiding violence and through conflict resolution reducing the level of intergroup disagreements, promoting physical and mental health – these and other steps will lead to law abiding behavior and reduce crime. The victims of crime lose their QOL.

Battered Women

Domestic violence against women is a worldwide problem that detracts greatly women and children's QOL. Studies in the United States, Australia, Sweden, Norway, and other countries have chiefly questioned women living in shelters, many of whom suffered abuse from their spouses for years, sometimes up to a decade or more, before leaving the household and seeking security and protection. Many women were unemployed and did not have adequate support for themselves and their children. Administrators of shelters conceal the location to prevent further abuse.

Acts of violence against women in domestic situations may be preceded by threats, threats to kill, threats to take children away, and other menaces. Acts of violence may include striking the head, beating, choking, forcing the woman to have sexual intercourse against her will, etc. Men committing these acts often are intoxicated. In addition to bodily pain, the victims suffer psychological, sexual, and social remorse, which often continues after removal to a shelter. Employed women are more likely to leave a threatening domestic situation.

In the Norway study (Alsker, Moen, & Kristoffersen, 2008), battered women in shelters were followed up 1 year after entering the shelter. It found that leaving the abusive partner improved the woman's QOL. Less improvement in the QOL was observed in women who had suffered greater abuse. Those who reported higher levels of abuse also suffered subsequently greater stress, depression, and physical health problems. Women found benefit in the security and social support the shelter offered; it helped to reduce their feelings of depression and anxiety. Women with a support network or with financial resources fared better after leaving an abusive partner. Unemployment remains a problem for many after entering a shelter.

In a study by Rokach (2006), two samples of women, an abused group ($n = 80$) and a general population of women ($n = 84$), were compared on a number of psychological characteristics. Abused women cope with loneliness more successfully than other women. In this condition, shelter workers may help them begin self-development practices, make new friends, and revive former friendships. Enrolling in self-development courses also is a possibility. Comparing the two samples shows that abused women would be amenable to and benefit from religious practices. The study found that abused women's tendency to cope with loneliness provides a key to their understanding of themselves and helps them better adjust to their life circumstances.

Shelters provide helpful security for battered women. Employment and childcare services are needed to facilitate their return to normality.

Summary of Steps to Maintain Order

A worldwide problem in the twenty-first century is the reduction of violence. Hate groups and terrorist organizations shatter the order and security of nations and communities. Military and police action to apprehend the perpetrators is required.

Conflicts based upon class, upon religious differences, and also upon cultural inconsistencies generate terroristic activities that destroy peace and tranquility. Practicing tolerance for others, teaching it in schools, and advocating it through public figures, media, and leaders appears to be the best solution. Consideration of others, especially, is needed in marital relations. Violence to destroy the opponent is not a solution.

This chapter and others have outlined steps that support the conservative position. Taking steps herein outlined on abiding by the tenants of a free-market society, cultivating attitudes and beliefs supportive of the community, becoming creative in intellectual or artistic pursuits, acting on behalf of a clean and toxin-free environment, avoiding violence through conflict resolution, reducing the level of intergroup disagreements, and promoting physical and mental health – these and other steps would reduce crime and improve security. However, the problem of reducing violence and ensuring safety continues. It requires vigilance and concerted governmental action and will not be solved quickly. Improving the QOL depends upon it.

Chapter 8
Hierarchy

> *The love of wealth is therefore to be traced, as either a principal*
> *or accessory motive, at the bottom of all that the Americans do;*
> *this gives to all their passions a sort of family likeliness . . . . It*
> *may be said that it is the vehemence of their desires that makes*
> *the Americans so methodical; it perturbs their minds, but it*
> *disciplines their lives.*
> Alexis de Tocqueville (1835), Democracy in America, Third
> Book, Chap. 1

> In battle or business, whatever the game,
> In law or in love, it is ever the same;
> In the struggle for power, or the scramble for pelf,
> Let this be your motto, – Rely on yourself!
> For, whether the prize be a ribbon or throne,
> The victor is he who can go it alone.
> *–John Godfrey Saxe, The Game of Life, Stanza 7*

Hierarchy. Distinctions of wealth, social power, authority, usually based upon material prosperity, social actualization, material well-being.

Proposition 8. The QOL may be enhanced through reducing the low-income segment of the population, minimizing distinctions based upon power and authority, improving the material well-being of the community, and expanding opportunities for community service and chances to achieve economic well-being.

Stratification

Power and authority are distributed unequally in society. In some societies, the arrangement is pyramidal, with a few at the top with much power and many at the bottom with little. Conversely, some societies are organized more equitably, with power and authority held by different individuals for different purposes: for labor, for religion, for production of goods or services, for governing, etc. Some societies, especially small primitive ones, have minimal structure, with a few individuals holding authority over segments, such as food, or spiritual concerns, or relations with other tribes. Thus, the social structure of the society dictates the hierarchy and an individual's position in it. Layers of strata characterize most societies.

A.L. Ferriss, *Approaches to Improving the Quality of Life*, Social Indicators Research
Series 42, DOI 10.1007/978-90-481-9148-2_8, © Springer Science+Business Media B.V. 2010

The strata one occupies, one's rank, affect one's motive to work. One strives to maintain one's position or to move up in rank. The system thus rewards individuals for their contributions: in money, power, or authority. These rewards give satisfaction and contribute to the person's QOL. Society functions and changes through the strata of power and authority.

Those living in a primitive culture may identify several power positions, based upon wealth or political power or age, but otherwise consider everyone equal. As an example in a more advanced culture, the Russian communist system attempted to eliminate the traditional Russian class hierarchy and instead gave members of the Communist Party special status. The Party granted distinctions and privileges to those of high rank in the Party.

In addition to power and authority, societies are also stratified by other traits. A generation may inherit its social rank position from the preceding generation. Occupation may be used as an indicator of status, with professional and technical workers at the top and common laborers and farm laborers at the bottom. Education may also distinguish strata, with those with the most years of education at the top, or the highest degree, scaling down to those with little formal education. Income also provides a stratified gradient, and so does wealth. A society may rank families according to their traditional position, no matter what their current education, wealth, or power is. Since these indicators of rank are correlated, some studies combine them into a socioeconomic status index (SES). People are motivated to move higher in the rank order, thus improving their position and their QOL. Or, they may adjust to their rank and remain content.

Social Class

Societies are structured into strata, reinforced by cultural definitions and values. Persons in strata have common interests with one another, those with common interests comprising a class. A class has its own values that define the good life, the desirable qualities of the QOL. This explains why some who live in much reduced physical and environmental conditions find the condition satisfying and fulfilling, whereas a member of another class might consider such conditions intolerable.

A social class may possess power and political influence. It may be distinguished by the educational attainment of its members, the education representing some special skill and knowledge held by its members, such as medical knowledge or architectural skill. Finally, wealth and income may demarcate and distinguish groups as separate classes. These distinctions provide the class identity: inheritance, social status, political power, education, and wealth.

Societies differ in the extent of class differences. Some have few class distinctions, while others have many levels, each with its own aura of honor and power. For our interest, the living conditions of the class provide an indicator of the QOL of the class – the size and location of the house, the type of automobile, and the like.

Some cultures emphasize skin color or other physiological features as a distinguishing feature of class. Ethnic status leads to class assignment by the society. These features may lead to a caste system, as exists in India.

Mobility from one class position to another, whether upward to a higher status or downward, may affect the movers' QOL. Social systems differ in whether free movement from class to class is allowed, some being more open than others.

Following Karl Marx, modern theorists have postulated four classes, based upon the relation of class position to the means of production. Capitalists own the means of production; managers control the labor of others for the owners; laborers have their strength and sweat to offer; and finally, the petty bourgeoisie own small enterprises employing a few workers. Rather than rigorous class lines, most theorists settle for a ranking of positions on a ladder. Some theorists, such as C. Wright Mills, conclude that modern conditions have decreased the importance of class, that the social system is more homogeneous.

Following Max Weber, recent scholars have posited property, prestige, and power as defining class position. This acknowledges the dominance of bureaucratic organizations in modern society. Occupational skills influence power/party position and contribute to one's social position. One owns property and that, also, influences one's position in society.

Class distinctions in the United States are difficult to identify, for income and occupational status are not straightforwardly related. Neither does educational attainment signify income level. In the end, economic status coupled with occupation do much to identify tastes, preferences, attitudes, and values which a member of a class may entertain in achieving its QOL.

The beginning grades in school are formative of future class position, for the quality of instruction and the class performance of the student determine subsequent academic position. Currently, in the United States, females are out-performing males in schools. Some immigrant children are excelling, in particular, those from Asia. Many children of Hispanic or African background underperform. These differences will resonate later in life, when educational achievement will influence class position.

One's social class position conditions social relations with others. Whether these relationships are satisfying or not contributes to the QOL. The class position one holds – one's power position – affects these relations.

To be admired socially becomes a source of satisfaction. Being upwardly mobile or downwardly mobile in the class structure influences others' evaluation of an individual.

Homelessness

Homelessness represents the nadir of material well-being. Examining the reasons for it may suggest bases for reducing and eliminating it. Ami Rokach (2004) compared responses of 266 homeless persons with 595 men and women from the general population of a Canadian city. The inability of the homeless to secure their basic needs leads to stress, a sense of inadequacy, and failure. Comparisons of the responses of the homeless with those of the general population led the author to identify the following as causes of the homeless condition: they feel personally inadequate that they do not "fit in." They sense deficits in their home/family relationships, feeling rejected by their family. Similarly, they feel they had unfulfilling personal relationships with their partner at home, some feeling emotionally abused, which, for some, may have led to a complete breakdown in intimate relationships. Having left home, they sense isolation and a loss of emotional support. Further assaults on their sensibilities accrue as a result of being arrested as a vagrant, being incarcerated, and suffering unemployment. The homeless also suffer from others' lack of trust in them because of being arrested, etc. The homeless female, particularly, lacks fulfilling intimate relationships.

From these results, it appears that relationships within the family and home lead to departure of the persons who eventually becomes lonely and homeless.

Another student of homelessness has identified contributing factors: as mental illness, autism and related disorders that impair living at home with others, and substance abuse. The solution to the problem must lie in the home. There, relationships among members require civility, sympathy, empathy, etc., to create bonds that hold individuals together. Social workers and family advisers need to find ways to build such relationships in families beset by conflict and friction. Mental illness, discussed in Chapter 2, deters a satisfying QOL.

The Lower Segment

The World Bank estimates that of the 6.2 billion people in the world, perhaps 2.5 billion of them survive on $2.00 a day or less. This represents a worldwide problem to confront homelessness, hunger, and lack of productive employment. Nonetheless, during the past 40 years, some countries have significantly improved their per capita income. Among them are Botswana, Brazil, China, Hong Kong, Indonesia, Japan, South Korea, Malaysia, Malta, Oman, Singapore, Taiwan, Thailand, South Korea, and others. Living conditions can be improved.

Elements of success include attracting foreign investments and opening the country to foreign trade. Governments committed to economic growth are more successful when their politics are stable. About one-fourth of national income should go into saving or investment in productive enterprises. Inflation should be kept under control. The government should shoulder its responsibilities for maintaining economic stability, as the United States did during the 1980s and 1990s by adjusting interest rates. The government, also, should allow a free market to allocate resources and take steps to satisfy needs. In the end, an unfettered free market for commercial transactions should be the rule.

In our rapidly changing environment, societies need to adopt new inventions and technologies. For example, in a very short time the cell phone has become almost universally accepted throughout the world. New ideas are now transmitted rapidly. Globalization, whereby countries are not isolated from one another but maintain vigorous trade and communication, has become the economic mode of operation. Under these conditions, change is universal. Countries in need of better living conditions cannot depend entirely upon outside help. Internally, they must initiate programs to improve housing, infrastructure such as roads and public buildings, public health, the distribution of goods and services, and education. The critical element is finding ways to improve the QOL of the country. These steps may impinge upon the hierarchy of the country, enlarging the middle class and decreasing poverty. Globalization, the introduction of new inventions, improvement of the social structure of a country – these steps in modernization will improve the QOL.

Summary

The social structure of a social system may change as its middle class expands, as people move into large cities, and as its infrastructure improves. In accepting technological innovations, people are joining hands to accept change. With the modern capacity to create wealth through international trade and manufacturing, nations' first priority should be the reduction of widespread poverty. More than any other step, this would improve the world's QOL.

Chapter 9
Egalitarian Commitment

> *Man's capacity for justice makes democracy possible, but man's inclination to injustice makes democracy necessary.*
> —Reinhold Niebuhr, The Children of Light and the Children of Darkness

> The fateful question of the human species seems to me to be whether and to what extent the cultural process developed in it will succeed in mastering the derangements of communal life caused by the human instinct of aggression and self-destruction .... Men have brought their powers of subduing the forces of nature to such a pitch that by using them they could now very easily exterminate one another to the last man.
> —*Sigmund Freud, Civilization and Its Discontents*

> We hold these truths to be self-evident; that all men are created equal; that they are endowed by their creator with certain unalienable rights; that among these are life, liberty and the pursuit of happiness; that to secure these rights, governments are instituted among men, deriving their just powers from the consent of the governed; that whenever any form of government becomes destructive of these ends, it is the right of the people to alter or to abolish it, and to institute new government, laying its foundation on such principles, and organizing its powers in such form, as to them shall seem most likely to effect their safety and happiness.
> —*Thomas Jefferson, The Declaration of Independence*

Egalitarian Commitment. Equality, social justice, freedom, having positive relations with others regardless of social status, social acceptance, being part of a community, participating.

Proposition 9. The QOL may be enhanced by monitoring human rights violations and infringement upon one's civil liberties, and by augmenting equality and social justice, expanding positive relations with others, and incorporating civic groups into the social life of the community.

Civil Liberties

The civil authority that holds the value equality in its eyes stands high in achieving equitable QOL for all. In times of national emergency, the government may jeopardize civil rights or civil hate groups because of economic, political, or cultural prejudice. The QOL may suffer from the removal of civil liberties during war, owing

A.L. Ferriss, *Approaches to Improving the Quality of Life*, Social Indicators Research
Series 42, DOI 10.1007/978-90-481-9148-2_9, © Springer Science+Business Media B.V. 2010

to the fear that the presence of the enemy-related group may threaten national security. This was the case of the US Japanese citizens during World War II. The rights of ethnic Japanese were violated by the government. Years later, the government gave reparations to those offended. Even so, the government had damaged the QOL of the ethnic Japanese. Whatever the basis for the impingement, when one's civil rights are violated, the community suffers loss of its QOL.

Economic factors also may cause the government to violate civil liberties and damage a group's equalitarian status. Ethnic or status groups separated by economic inequality may give rise to violence and agitation. Labor unions have agitated against corporate management. An unemployed ethnic group may excite violence against the group it targets as threatening its jobs.

A group may justify a cultural meme, such as prejudice, against another group, and feel justified in violence against another group. The native group looks down upon the despised group because it is "different," with patterns of behavior of which the native group disapproves. The native group impinges upon the strange group's civil liberties, thus diminishing its QOL.

The American Civil Liberties Union (ACLU), established in 1920, defends violations of the liberties granted under the US Constitution, especially the 19 amendments. With over 500,000 members and supporters, ACLU has offices in nearly every state and handles some 6,000 court cases annually. As a guardian of American rights, ACLU publishes a variety of accounts of its activities, including human rights, free speech, HIV/AIDS, disability rights, death penalty, lesbian and gay rights, police practices, rural justice, privacy and technology, reproductive freedom, rights of the poor, voting rights, women's rights, safely and free of charge. Currently, it is stepping into the issue of the Guantanamo military mission where foreigners, suspected of being enemy combatants, are held without charges. As the watchdog alert to violations of constitutional rights, ACLU works to ensure egalitarian commitment for an environment to provide a better QOL.

Other organizations also are concerned with civil rights and their violation by hate groups. They include B'nai B'rith and the Southern Poverty Law Center.

Southern Poverty Law Center

The Southern Poverty Law Center of Montgomery, Alabama, USA, keeps track of hate groups active across the United States. In 2007, it identified 844 hate groups in the United States. A year later, there were 926 hate groups. For over 140 years, the Ku Klux Klan, now some 165 units strong, has engaged in lynching, bombing, rape, and other means of intimidation against blacks, Jews, Catholics, homosexuals, and various immigrant groups.

Some 191 neo-Nazi groups have arisen, creating hatred against Jews, and committing robberies, beatings, and murders. Some 78 racist skinhead organizations operate in small crews, with various targets that may involve illegal drugs and threats. At least 37 Christian identity groups spread hatred against Jews, hold non-whites to be "soulless mud people," and some believe Christ will not come again until Jews are exterminated.

Some 102 neo-Confederate groups are imbued with Civil War ideology, embracing racist attitudes and hoping for eventual Southern secession. One hundred and ten white nationalist groups seek to advance the white "race" against others, emphasizing the inferiority of non-whites and espousing white separatist ideas.

Blacks also have hate groups. They oppose the integration of blacks into the social system. Eighty-eight black separatist groups are anti-white and anti-Semitic; they seek to sponsor separate black institutions and geographic areas. In addition, there are 73 general hate groups that identify themselves as Blood and Honor, the Racial Nationalist Party of America, and Volksfront. Many are anti-government and violent.

The Southern Poverty Law Center has found that these groups are growing, a 40% increase from 2000 to 2006. The increase is partly due to aggression of hate groups against recent immigrants. These groups are less prevalent in the Great Plains and Mountain States but more prevalent in the East, especially South Carolina and New Jersey.

The Center assisted in legal action against two Klan members who, at a Kentucky fair, brutally beat Jordan Gruver, a 16-year-old US citizen of Panamanian Indian ancestry, whom the Klan members mistook for a Hispanic immigrant. The two Klan members pleaded guilty and were sentenced to 3 years in prison.

Thus, by taking legal action against hate group members, the Southern Poverty Law Center counteracts and in some cases eliminates hate groups. In the 1980s and 1990s, the Center sued Ku Klux Klan groups because of their aggression against African Americans. It won multimillion dollar judgments. Several Klans were forced into bankruptcy (Dees, 2007; Parker, 2007). The United Klans of America and the White Aryan Resistance went out of business.

Morris Dees, the chief council for SPLC, and associates filed suits in September 2000 against a Richard Butler, founder of Aryan Nations organization. The legal team won a 6.3 million dollar judgment, forcing the sale of Butler's 20-acre compound in Idaho. The Aryan Nations personnel and activities are described in a recently published book *Into the Devil's Den* (Ballantine Books). It recounts experiences of David Hall, an FBI informant who spent two and a half years with Aryan Nations. Plots to kill Morris Dees or attack the SPLC have resulted in more than 30 persons being incarcerated.

The work of the SPLC shows that a key to reducing such illegal attacks is through the court system, via legal action.

B'nai B'rith International

B'nai B'rith International has the mission of advancing human rights for Jews and others around the world. It actively champions the State of Israel. It has opposed an Arab boycott of Israel, international embargoes on Israeli military, academic, and scientific institutions, and business interests. It supports efforts to assist Jewish college youth and seniors with needs for affordable housing and medical care. It works in dozens of countries promoting human rights and opposing anti-Semitism. It maintains a website at www.bnaibrith.org.

Social Capital

Maximizing a person's social capital enhances the person's QOL. Social capital refers to the network of associations and relationships one has in the community, including trust, commitment, and communication. One calls upon one's network of associates to help accomplish a task or attain some other objective. The extent of such an informal network is one's social capital. When one's social capital leads to achieving greater satisfaction in accomplishments, one gains in QOL (Heinsohn, 2001).

Using the 2001 Quality of Work Life Survey of Spain, Requena (2003) found that higher levels of social capital generate higher levels of job satisfaction and quality of work life. A model that included personal variables, corporate variables of the work environment, family setting, and social capital variables achieved an R^2 of 0.59. He found that relationships of trust, communication, and so forth that stand for social capital generate higher levels of job satisfaction and quality of work life. He concluded, "Trust, social relations on the job, commitment to the company or organization, communication and possibilities of influence are all elements that explain a large portion of the total variance of satisfaction and quality of life in the workplace" (p. 356).

The concept is relatively new and is still evolving. Tarja Nieminen et al. (2008) identified various interpretations of the concept. With no thought of money, the World Bank, for example, measures social capital in six domains: "(1) groups and networks; (2) trust and solidarity; (3) collective action and cooperation; (4) information and communication; (5) social cohesion and inclusion; and (6) empowerment and political action." This, indeed, broadens the concept.

Nieminen et al. (2008) in a study identify four levels of participation (community, family, friends, etc.) and four elements of social capital (trust, tolerance, etc.) The United Kingdom Office of National Statistics employs five areas consisting of measures of participation and communication.

Employing data ($n = 8,028$) from the Finnish Health 2000 Survey and entering 39 variables reflecting social capital dimensions, a factor analysis resulted in four dimensions: trust, social support, and two social participation domains. The author found a high level of social capital among the rich, well-educated, young, and married, indicating their high QOL. The study suggested that social services to improve the social capital of the borderline persons who were excluded socially might be provided.

A Canadian study (Ravanera, 2007) found that married men living with children enjoyed higher social capital than lone fathers, step-fathers in cohabiting unions, or child-free men. The presence of children appears to contribute to the social capital of the husband and the family.

A network of associates must trust one another to accomplish anything. An indicator of the level of social capital in a community is the extent of voluntary association. Studies have shown an increase in such association in Germany, the Netherlands, Canada, and the United States. This means that citizens are voluntarily contributing to the welfare of the community and broadening trust and communication. These activities tend toward improving the community QOL and hence the QOL of individual participants. With a sample of 50 countries, Helliwell (2007) found social capital to improve life satisfaction as well as to reduce suicide rates.

With a sample of college students in Italy, Iran, and the United States, social participation was found to be correlated with Sense of Community and Identification with Community. (Cicognani et al., 2008) "Social participation positively affects social well-being through the mediation of Sense of Community" (p. 109). The college students, by country, exhibited different levels of participation in the community, but all showed positive with well-being. The study expanded the idea of Social Well-Being to include perceived social integration, social contribution (to the community), social acceptance (see Chapter 2, Social Acceptance), social actualization, and social coherence. The authors distinguished these from psychological aspects of well-being. Together, these features reinforce the Social Capital dimension of well-being. They support the idea that stimulating social participation leads to a higher QOL.

The impact of social capital on economic development in Europe was investigated by Isabel Neira, Vazquez, and Portela (2009). Using trust and membership in voluntary groups as indicators of social capital, they found social capital to be larger in Scandinavian countries and Western Europe than in Eastern Europe. The study investigated the effect social capital had upon economic development and concluded human and social capital had a positive impact. Despite the difficulties in measuring social capital, this result is significant, and prompts its inclusion in studies of development that traditionally consider employment and investment.

Another example of social capital is the network of relationships involved in small business loan enterprises. Usually administered by a group of women operating like a bank, these organizations issue small loans to support local economic enterprises. The lenders trust the recipients of the loans and monitor the enterprise until the loan is paid. By keeping trust, the recipient may receive a subsequent loan, building his/her social capital of trust. (See Chapter 3, Mastery, on Small Business Loans.)

A disaster caused by the accidental release of toxins in the air or an accidental spilling of an industrial waste, termed a technological disaster, is likely to diminish social capital. It reduces trust in the security of the community and creates uncertainty. On the other hand, a natural disaster, such as a cyclone, is likely to bring citizens together to assist one another and hence to increase social capital (Bonikowski & McPherson, 2007; Ritchie & Gill, 2007).

Bjornskov (2008) traced happiness and social capital indices for the United States from 1983 to 1998. His measures of happiness and social capital declined over the period. However, he found social trust and other social capital measures positively associated with happiness, an indicator of QOL. Across the American states and over time, trust is strongly associated with happiness. He says, "(C)ausality runs from social trust to happiness" (p. 56). In cross-sectional analysis of the American states, informal sociability is not significantly linked with happiness, and formal sociability is significant and negatively associated with happiness. Bjornskov calls for more study of these variables.

In seeking ways to improve community QOL, we should look for means for increasing social capital, to expand volunteerism and trust, and reduce social inequalities, thereby expanding equalitarian commitment.

Social Cohesion

This important group characteristic has been identified as one of four conditions needed for European QOL. The concept has now been clarified by Chan and associates (2006). They define it as "a state of affairs concerning both the vertical and horizontal interactions among members of society as characterized by a set of attitudes and norms that includes trust, a sense of belonging and the willingness to participate and help, as well as their behavioral manifestations" (p. 290). Notice that trust is included here as also it is in the concept of social capital, but the authors point out that trust in the social capital context is at the individual and group levels while social cohesion is more of a societal concept. The authors list 15 questions they suggest to provide a measure of the term, including an item on trust, cooperation, belonging, pride of country, participation in community groups, helpfulness to neighbors, volunteer work, financial contributions, organizer activities, trust and confidence in community organizations, opinion on current affairs, signing petitions, and voting on local issues. Thus, social cohesion by their definition involves both vertical and horizontal interactions with societal activities. One would expect societies high in social cohesion to provide an environment conducive to the good life and a high level of the QOL.

Civil Rights

The General Assembly of the United Nations, in 1945, established the Universal Declaration of Human Rights. Through its Office of the High Commissioner for Human Rights, it monitors and investigates violations of human rights worldwide. Information on its activities is available from its website, www.ohchr.org.

Amnesty International is a non-governmental organization that investigates and initiates action against violations of human rights worldwide. It assembles information on violations of human rights, seeking to expose them and bring about redemptive action. It has identified humanitarian and human rights problems in the Democratic Republic of the Congo, Darfur, Gaza and southern Israel, and other locations. It also has exposed violations against the rights of women, reporting that such violations in some countries affect some 70% of women. It prompts the United Nations to act against violence toward civilians suffering starvation and disease and to deploy UN peacekeepers to areas of conflict, it seeks to bring perpetrators that violate civil rights to justice, and it promotes peace in war-torn areas, such as Sudan.

In South Africa, whites violated the civil rights of black natives for generations. When blacks eventually gained control, their rights were legally restored. A Truth and Recollection Commission, guided by former Archbishop Desmond Tutu, brought contending sides together, completing its work in 1998. Under democracy, the people obtained freedom of movement. Many migrated into the cities. These and other achievements have marked a movement toward egalitarian society, though much remains to be accomplished (Moller, 2007).

Immigrants to the United States have come in waves that have sometimes generated opposition by residents. The strangers bring different cultural values and behavior patterns, and the natives do not immediately accept them. In some instances, they have rioted to express anger at their treatment, as also have citizens, for perceived infringement on their rights. The country has not always been peaceful.

In 1886, workers rioted for an 8-h day of work in Haymarket, Chicago. Eleven people died. In 1863, during the Civil War, draft riots in New York City resulted in about 1,000 fatalities. In 1908, Springfield, IL, witnessed an anti-black riot. In 1943, during World War II, in Detroit, a race riot left 34 dead and 700 injured, while in New York City, six were killed in the Harlem section. In 1965, at the time of racial disturbances, 34 deaths resulted from a riot in the Watts section of Los Angeles, with much property damage. The year 1967 was fraught with trouble. In Newark, NJ, 26 were killed and some 1,500 injured, while in Detroit, rioting, looting, and other action resulted in 43 deaths and some 2,000 being injured in black neighborhoods. Los Angeles was again the scene of riot against the police, resulting in 52 deaths. Violation of civil rights and other infringements have resulted in these incidences of disorder.

Far more devastating to civil liberties of the strangers has been the antagonism of hate groups against African Americans, Hispanics, and other minorities. In employing aggression and rioting, groups have destroyed for the moment their QOL. The philosophy of peaceful protest, espoused by Martin Luther King, Jr., who was influenced by Mohandas Gandhi, offers a more nonviolent way to bring about social change. (The figures in this section are estimates of fatalities from newspaper accounts.)

Reconciliation

To reduce the animosity between racial groups, nations, and people who have enmity toward one another, religious bodies have pursued programs of reconciliation. One such program arose from the bombing of Coventry, England, during World War II. The resulting charred cross of nails has become a worldwide symbol, generating harmony between formerly hostile groups. Some 160 centers around the world work for peace and harmony within their communities and countries. With a religious orientation, the groups "are committed to praying for reconciliation." There are no boundaries, neither conceptual nor personal, to the program, which embodies "politics, race, religion, economics, sexual orientation, or personal." Cross of Nails centers are in South Africa, Nigeria, Burundi, Israel, and Palestine, the United States (43 centers), Germany, Northern Ireland, and other locations. The centers provide motivation, leadership, and inspiration to foster understanding and trust between previously hostile entities.

Another effort arises from the philosophy of the late Martin Luther King, Jr. The Southern Christian Leadership Conference opened two centers in the Middle East that promote nonviolence and reconciliation. Also involved is the Center for Non-Violence and Peace Studies of the University of Rhode Island. A center in Bethlehem and one in Dimona, Israel, provide nonviolence training to local people. During the past 15 years, two of the leaders, Charles Alphin and Bernard Lafayette, have promoted the idea of nonviolent change in Haiti, Columbia, India, and the Soviet Union. The Middle East program provides instruction in nonviolence action to social workers, political leaders, and activists across the West Bank and Gaza Strip. The nonviolence philosophy has led to beneficial change in India and the United States. It holds promise to engender change via peaceful solutions to conflict situations in the Middle East, to the eventual improvement in the QOL.

Human Rights

In 1948, the Universal Declaration of Human Rights set forth a definition, "all human beings are born free and equal in dignity and rights. They are endowed with conscience and should act towards one another in a spirit of brotherhood." Recently, the UN Human Rights Council has been organized to look into violations.

A perspective on violations would first designate the layer of social structure, the specific group whose human rights are being violated, and also identify the aggressors. What is the rationale for the aggression? Is there an economic basis? Are jobs at risk? Or is there cultural animosity between the groups? A different lifestyle, perhaps? The manner of aggression should be identified, whether street marching, setting fire to a building, aggression against churches, haranguing to voice anger and prejudice, or the use of symbols, such as burning a cross. Further analysis would identify the action against the hate group, such as court action or police intervention.

Countries differ in the degree to which women are accepted in various economic and social statuses. Gender inequality has been studied by Tesch-Romer, Motel-Kingebiel, and Tomasik (2008). Findings from the World Values Survey, involving 57 countries, reveal wide country differences in the treatment of women. Countries were classified according to whether they agreed or disagreed with the statement that when jobs are scarce, men should have greater priority in employment than women. Countries accepting gender inequality on the labor market were negatively correlated with subjective health and life satisfaction. In contrast, countries rejecting gender inequality were positively correlated with subjective health and life satisfaction. The study presents strong evidence for the liberation of women in the workplace, in order to improve their health and QOL.

Liberation, also, of lesbian women and gay men (LGB) has become a concern in the United States. Recent decades have shown increasing acceptance of LGB in the workplace. A recent small-sample interview study has uncovered problems they face. These involve stereotyping, gender discrimination, and sexual harassment (Giuffre, Dellinger, & Williams, 2008). Stereotyping involves heterosexuals questioning LGBs concerning aspects of their sexuality. This may lead to isolating them. It also may lead to harassment on the (false) grounds of "converting" LGBs to heterosexuality. Stereotyping also involves gender inversion in their treatment, based upon the assumed dual nature of the condition. The study implied that treatment of LGBs in the workplace would be more equitable if more than one were present. Most workplaces promote a monogamous, nuclear family, heterosexual ideal. Most LGBs do not conform to this ideal. LGBs must repress or hide their emotions in order to be accepted. Another problem arises due to the current legal restriction on any sexual harassment in the workplace. Based upon interviews with the sample of LGBs, the study contends that it is important to allow workers to respond to both wanted and unwanted sexual interests. Gender discrimination may be modified by recognizing and rewarding qualities associated with femininity, whether present in men or women. These are tentative observations of the study, requiring more extensive consideration of LGB experience and concerns, but they point to steps that may reduce inequity suffered by LGBs, and enhance their QOL.

There are a number of organizations working for the reduction of human rights violations. In addition to the efforts of organizations described above, there are many others, including Sociologists Without Borders, Rights Works International, and the Columbia University Center for the Study of Human Rights.

Social Change and Anomie

Groups that have been deprived of their rights may find improvement by change in social structure of the social system. Change in structure may come about as a result of revolution, peaceful change in the political system, or some economic transformation brought about by technological innovation. Whatever the cause, an alteration in social structure affects the QOL of subgroups.

The theory of this study is that the socio-economic-cultural system affects the QOL, and changes in the system are required to improve the QOL. One debilitating result of change often is a condition of *anomie.*

With the breakdown of the socialist system in Eastern Europe, the political and economic systems assumed the Western open-market model, leading to change in norms and orientations. For a time, a lack of understanding arose, creating normlessness and powerlessness. Individuals had difficulty keeping up with the pace of social change. A condition of *anomie* affected subgroups in Eastern Europe. *Anomie* is a condition of powerlessness, an absence of societal guidance in the form of norms. The norms of the social system do not support the individual, and previously held meanings no longer apply. Studies have shown a rise in anomie in these countries and a lower QOL. As time has brought about better understanding, conditions have improved and anomie has declined. Studies from 1999 to 2002 have shown the Czech Republic and East Germany to have lower anomie.

South Africa underwent vast social change with the rise of control by Blacks and Coloreds (South African term for mixed race and Asian peoples) and the decline of the influence of Whites in the political, but not the economic, sphere. In 1994, with the election of Blacks, great enthusiasm for the new order generated optimism among the Blacks, but concern among some Whites. As time went on, health clinics, clean water, and electricity were improved, but housing, employment, income, and living conditions did not improve immediately. Social inequalities remained. Whites, on the other hand, reported themselves happy but were pessimistic about the future. Blacks showed the highest level of anomie, while Whites showed significantly less. Thus, happiness and satisfaction with life are associated with the level of anomie. The authors of this analysis, Huschka and Mau (2006), attribute low educational levels of Blacks as hindering the integration of Blacks into the institutional framework of South Africa. To adjust to the new, Blacks need to understand the "new political, administrative, social and judicial systems." The aspects of anomie – "social isolation, normlessness, self-estrangement and powerlessness" – need to be overcome. The result will be an improved QOL.

Morality

One's sense of morality prompts empathy for others, sympathy, and civil behavior. How do we acquire morality? Moral behavior, sympathetic actions for another's misfortune, and other evidence of empathy have been observed among higher apes. Frans de Waal (2006) has shown that chimpanzees and other higher apes exhibit moral behavior in their relations with their kind. The notable incident in a zoo illustrates apes' morality. A 3-year-old boy had fallen into a gorilla's enclosure. The gorilla, Binta Jua, rescued the boy and carried him in her arms to the door of her cage, so that zoo-keepers could take care of him.

In addition to the possible genetic basis for moral behavior among humans, humans acquire morality through social relationships and culture. They learn group norms through a socialization process that involves imitation, status attainment, and sanctions for violation of norms. Violation may prompt various forms of discipline, such as shunning or disfellowshipping (a term used by Jehovah's Witnesses), or other enforcement strategies.

Distributive Justice

Being a victim of a crime diminishes one's QOL. Crime imposes costs without a corresponding reward. Crime sometimes stimulates fear, despondency, and even death, the final cost. Having one's purse snatched or one's pocket picked happens annually to 116 of 1,000 persons 12 years of age and older. The next most frequent US crime is having one's house burglarized. Nearly 30 persons of 1,000 a year suffer house burglary. Victims pay the cost in lost property, suffer emotional strain, and lose to some degree trust in their fellow man. About 18 of 1,000 persons are assaulted, often being injured physically. Bringing the perpetrator of these crimes to justice and imposing punishment does not restore the cost to the victim, even though it may restore order to society to some degree. Social control and protection of individuals and the community within the limits of law stands as the goal of the system of police, courts, and detention facilities. Security of the individual leads to a better QOL.

Religious Radicalism

In a Dallas, TX, trial of the Holy Land Foundation involving the extremist Muslim Brotherhood (Ikhwan), the FBI introduced a 1991 document outlining a plan for destroying Western Civilization and establishing rule by a global Islamic state governed by Sharia. The attack of September 11, 2001, was viewed as part of the plan. According to the document, the jihad aims to destroy Western Civilization from within by radicalizing Muslim organizations such as the Council on American Islamic Relations, the Islamic Society of North America, and the Muslim-American Society. The goal is to make "God's religion ... victorious over all religions," according to documents introduced in the trial by the FBI. Dr. Zuhdi Jasser of the American Islamic Forum for Democracy has affirmed the intentions of radical Islam to take over Muslim institutions in the United States. Conserving American democratic institutions becomes a task for governmental security forces. Alert citizens must provide authorities with any information concerning this threat. American democratic institutions are culturally essential to its QOL.

Summary of Initiatives to Improve QOL

Taking legal action against hate groups is effective in curtailing hate.
Training police officers to identify members of hate groups.
Reconciliation through action of moral norms of organized groups.
Monitoring and combating anti-Semitic and other behaviors that impinge upon the rights of others, especially minorities, women, and homosexuals.
Supporting anti-hate, and anti-human rights groups.
Reducing crime through improving police and other security agencies.
Improving economic conditions of the poor through small-enterprise loans.
Reinforcing norms of morality and justice in the community.
Expanding the social capital of persons in communities through maximizing participation and reducing fear.

Chapter 10
Health

Look to your health; and if you have it, praise God,
and value it next to a good conscience; for health
is the second blessing that we mortals are capable of,
a blessing that money cannot buy.
> – *Izaak Walton, The Compleat Angler, Chap. XXI*

(In a state of nature) No arts, no letters, no society,
and, which is worst of all, continual fear and danger
of violent death, and the life of man solitary, poor, nasty,
brutish, and short.
> – *Thomas Hobbes, Leviathan, Chap. XIII*

Yes, death is at the bottom of the cup,
And every one that lives must drink it up;
And yet between the sparkle at the top
And the black lees where lurks that bitter drop,
There swims enough good liquor, Heaven knows,
To ease our hearts of all their other woes.
> – *William Dean Howells, If.*

Always free I must
Dart light-headedly from joy to joy
I want my life to glide
Along the paths of pleasure,
Whether the day is born or dying,
Always gay at parties,
My thought must fly
Always to new delights.
> – *Giuseppe Verdi, La Traviata, Act I*

Health. Mental and physical well-being, physical vigor. Not only absence of disease and disability but a state of mental, physical, and social well-being. Low health is indicated by illness, lack of positive feelings, lack of exercise, excessive weight, etc.

Proposition 10. The QOL will be enhanced through reducing illness and disability and by improving the physical and mental health of the community through public health programs that encourage more nutritious food consumption, opportunities for regular exercise, rest and relaxation, and through attention to personal disabilities through medical care. Good health is a prime requirement of a flourishing QOL.

A.L. Ferriss, *Approaches to Improving the Quality of Life*, Social Indicators Research
Series 42, DOI 10.1007/978-90-481-9148-2_10, © Springer Science+Business Media B.V. 2010

Good health, as Izaak Walton tells us, is a basic requirement for well-being. It comes from obeying a few common rules or practices that promote vigor and mental health and by avoiding practices that cause disabilities. A long healthy life is the aim. Avoid the debilitating effects of tobacco, alcohol, toxins in the air, and overconsumption of proteins and fats. Exercise, eat fruits and vegetables, and maintain an optimistic attitude to enjoy healthy years and many of them. This text will focus primarily upon the means to good health, rather than medical practice to repair disabilities.

Using four measures of health, Michalos and Zumbo (2002) explained 17–28% of the variance in QOL satisfaction scores. They employed the Center for Disease Control and Prevention measures, which included the three healthy days variable, the not good physical health days variable, and the not good mental health days variable. With the health satisfaction variable included, some 40% of the variance in the QOL score was explained. Six surveys were conducted in Canada, including a British Columbia sample, one of Quesnel, three samples of Prince George, and one of Mackenzie. The result establishes firmly that health is an essential element in QOL measurement.

Socioeconomic Influences

Health is not evenly distributed in the population. Ethnic and socio-demographic factors distinguish population segments that suffer poorer health. This is owing to genetics, cultural tradition, occupation, gender, lifestyle, and other causes. Studies show that females in the United States are in worse health than are males, groups in some localities suffer environmental toxins, and white people have better health than do blacks or Hispanics. Educational attainment is associated with health status, those with less education being in poorer health. Employed persons report being in better health than others. Physical health becomes worse with age, but not mental health (Jai et al., 2007; Green, Kerstetter, & Nylander III, 2008).

Between 1960 and 1990, child mortality improved nearly two-fifths. The World Bank attributed the gains to improved education of women. Reading skill, also, affects health, owing to the need to read instructions, labels, and other medical instructions. In less-developed countries, low literacy levels hamper steps to improve health and the QOL. Poor people, as reflected in a country's GDP, suffer higher infant mortality and shorter life expectancy at birth. Conversely, a few countries with low GDP have a higher than expected life expectancy, Sri Lanka being one, with $810 GDP per capita but male and female life expectancy of 71 and 75 years, respectively, in a recent year. This suggests that increasing the income of a country will not inevitably improve health and that education, housing, sanitation, and health services also must be improved if health is to improve (Ratzam, Filerman, & Sar, 2000).

Persons with health insurance report better health than those with no insurance. There are also regional variations in health, skin cancer being greater in areas with more exposure to the sun's rays. Thus, environmental factors, occupational influences, age, gender, and ethnic status all influence behavior that may lead to adverse health conditions and illness, impacting the QOL.

Life Expectancy

During the twentieth century and to 2004, the life expectancy of males in the United States increased from 46.3 to 75.2 years and for females, from 48.3 to 80.4 years. Better treatment of infants, improved nutrition, medical care, public hygienic conditions, and housing have contributed to better QOL and longevity. In the more developed regions of the world, life expectancy at birth averages 76 years, while in less-developed areas, it is 67 years.

Japan and European countries exceed the United States in life expectancy. Japan's life expectancy at birth is 81 years compared with 77.8 (in 2004) for the United States. Other countries with longer life expectancy are Sweden, Switzerland, Italy, and Australia, each with 80 years, France, 79, and the United Kingdom, 78. At the other extreme stand African countries, Eastern African countries averaging 47 years life expectancy, Middle African countries averaging 49 years, and Southern Africa, 50 years. Infant mortality, malaria, and tuberculosis are the primary causes. These data are current to 2002. Social factors loom large in affecting the death rate.

Life expectancy in Italy, over the 1991–2000 period, found for men increases from 73.5 to 76 years and for women from 79.9 to 82.1 years. However, when disability-free life expectancy is considered, the female advantage in years is reduced, their QOL because of disability being greater than men's. Regional differences in Italy also exist. The southern region has worse quality of health than the central and northern regions. The study also found mental illness to exert a disabling influence on the QOL in Italy (Burgio, Murrianni, & Folino-Gallo, 2009).

Behavioral Risk Factor Surveillance System

A monthly sample survey of the United States shows that general life satisfaction is related negatively to mean unhealthy days. The Behavioral Risk Factor Surveillance System is a continuous state-by-state US survey that has produced annual estimates of health-related QOL matters since 1993. The Survey probes the past 30 days for the number of healthy and unhealthy days. The 1998 survey showed that the respondents with a mean of 3.5 unhealthy days during a month were very satisfied with life, while those very dissatisfied reported 19.1 mean unhealthy days. The US Survey over time shows unhealthy days increasing and people increasingly less satisfied with life. The trend from 1993 to 2001 shows mean unhealthy days of adults to have increased from approximately 5–6 days (Moriarty, 2007).

Health, according to the 1993–2001 surveys, is highly related to education and income, two measures indicative of QOL. Those reporting excellent health increased from 11% with less than high school education to 35% with college education. Those with less than $15,000 annual household income reported 14% excellent health, while those with more that $50,000 annual income reported 34% excellent health. At the other extreme in self-reported health, for those reporting fair or poor health, the opposite is true: 35% versus 6% for education and 32% versus 5% in income (Zahran et al., 2005).

It appears quite clear, then, that good health is an essential ingredient in good QOL.

Medical Technologies

Biotechnology is developing chemicals that enhance human capabilities. The future use of many of these chemicals is yet to be realized, but a number of organizations are anticipating that genetic engineering, drugs that stimulate the brain, and other means of biomedical enhancement are in the wave of the future. The San Francisco Institute for Global Futures, the National Institute of Biomedical Imaging and Bioengineering, Genentech, Inc., and others at various universities are probing future applications of chemicals for human enhancement. Some, however, are less confident. The President's Council on Bioethics in 2003 issued a report *Beyond Therapy* warning against too rapid acceptance of the new technologies. *Reproduction and Responsibility: The Regulation of New Technologies* (2004) explores this further. Government regulation may be required to control usage. The development of medical interventions to treat diseases, thus, is leading to medical technologies with the potential of improving the human condition.

A study at the University of Maryland found that college students (18% of a 1,208 sample) were taking medications such as Ritalin and Adderall to help concentration while studying, even through the medications had not been approved by the Food and Drug Administration for this purpose. "To improve concentration" is the reason given by others for taking prescription drugs that enhance concentration. In addition, the drugs are said to enhance attention, memory, and creativity (Baker, 2009). The drugs influence the brain chemicals dopamine and norepinephrine, which enhance memory and attention. Some of the research has shown that the drugs that affect the brain will slow the development of such diseases as Alzheimer's, Parkinson's, and Huntington's. Historical research has uncovered the use of hallucinogenic drugs by artists to enhance their creativity. Edvard Munch used drugs to help paint such masterpieces as "The Scream," and Vincent van Gogh saw rings around lights because of the digitalis he took for epilepsy. Research is also investigating the use of brain-enhancing electrical circuits. These and other results of recent research are reported in *Pharmacotherapy, Nature, Brain Waves, Pharmacological Research,* and similar journals (Baker, 2009).

Alternative Treatments

The National Institutes of Health created the National Center for Complementary and Alternative Medicine (phone: 888-644-6226). It has supported some 1,800 research projects at 260 institutions addressing integrative therapies. Alternative treatment strategies for persons with such debilitating illnesses as heart disease, cancer, and others are being practiced at medical institutions in almost every state. The integrated treatments include meditation (Tibetan meditation), yoga, music therapy, nutrition, exercise, acupuncture, healing touch, herbal therapy, and other treatments, generally termed integrative medicine. Results include a reduction in blood pressure, lower stress and depression, reduction of arterial restriction, and other benefits to the QOL. Medical professionals are admitting that Western medicine may be successfully supplemented by application of other healing systems. The gestalt of the patient is engaged. More information is available at www.nccam.nih.gov.

Some consider meditation, prayer, and faith to better control disease. The press reported a psychiatrist at the University of Miami, Dr. Gail Ironson, as holding this view. Dr. Andrew Newberg at the University of Pennsylvania also agrees. Those who attend religious services have been found to live longer than non-attendees, according to Hummer and associates (1999). Religious organizations offer social support – churches, synagogues, mosques (See Chapter 2). Fasting, with the notion of cleansing the body of toxins and the mind of past digressions, also has been used as a bridge to better health. Those who advise fasting insist that it be carried out under supervision of medical specialists. It has been found to benefit some health conditions, but not all (Fuhrman, 1999).

American teens transmit sexual diseases to one another at alarming rates. It is "The Hidden Epidemic," according to a report by the National Academy of Sciences' Institute of Medicine. Race plays a part. The rate of gonorrhea among African-Americans is 18 times greater than among whites. Only slightly less dramatic are rates for syphilis, chlamydial infection, and HIV-AIDS. Studies attribute concurrent sexual partnerships of more than one person at a time as contributing. Drug use through sharing needles also affects HIV-AIDS transmission. In this environment, treating one person at a time is ineffective. Experts are suggesting that sexual health of our youth become the basis for national discussion. Improvement of social conditions of poor neighborhoods and a change in sexual practices may mitigate the problem. While not 100%, the use of condoms provides some protection.

The Gallup Organization surveyed the US population daily during 2008 to ascertain the basis and condition of the good life. The Gallup – Healthways Well-Being Index, based upon 100,000 interviews, shows that 49% identify themselves as "thriving," while almost as many, 47%, characterize themselves as "struggling." The remaining 4% are "suffering." These are broad characterizations, of course, based upon the "ladder" that the Gallup interviewer asks the respondent to consider, zero being the lowest and ten the highest rungs. Those in the higher rungs of the ladder have better QOL, less illness, higher incomes, and better work environments than those in the lower rungs of the ladder.

The Gallup survey finds 89% of the US population feeling happy on the day prior to the interview, and 84% feeling "enjoyment." Some 38% acknowledged experiencing "stress" and 30% "worry." Physical pain (23%), sadness (17%), and anger (13%) represent experiences that deplete the QOL. The Gallup – Healthways Well-Being Index does not show a constant mood among Americans, but rather an oscillating one with four or five peaks each month, each peak followed by a nadir or low point. The low mood is always followed by an upturn. Information on these aspects of the QOL enables advances in understanding the social conditions affecting people. It could lead to more intelligent policies and programs to improve the QOL.

Mental Illness

Individuals' mental health state has been classified as flourishing, moderately mental healthy, or languishing. Approximately one-fifth of US adults aged 25–74 are judged to be flourishing. They are at lower risk of chronic physical disease and are more productive at work. Languishing individuals, however, functioned no better and sometimes worse than individuals in a depressed state of mental health. These and other results are from a special issue of *Social Indicators Research* (Keyes, 2006).

Some 3.1% of the US population over age 17 years suffer from serious psychological distress. The figure results from a six item scale from a household interview in 2002–2003. Poor people (8.7%) suffer greater distress than non-poor (1.8%). The Hispanic population suffers in slightly greater percentages (3.9) than the white (3.0). However, poor whites are affected by psychological distress to a much greater extent than any other category (10.1%). Young adults, 18–24 years, are less beset by mental illness (only 2.8%), but a peak is reached during the 45–54 years. The proportion mentally ill then declines with increasing age (National Center for Health Statistics, 2005).

These figures represent serious psychological distress. Many more, however, suffer depression and other mental illnesses that limit their QOL. Serious depression, for example, will affect 6.3% of the population – 19 million persons – at any one time, and at some time in their life, 16% of the US population will fall into depression. By affecting one's mood, thoughts, and feelings, depression dampens the QOL.

European countries vary widely in experiencing depressive symptoms. Eighteen percent of males and 26% of females report them. The rate of depression increases with age (Huppert et al., 2009). Norway, Denmark, and Switzerland – countries with high QOL – report very low levels of depression, while at the other extreme, high levels of depression prevail in Hungary, Ukraine, and Portugal: around 40%t. The European Social Survey reveals that people with depression report that they do not have time to do the things they enjoy doing, feel that they are not treated with respect, and do not do voluntary work. Perhaps if they did these things, their symptoms of depression would decline. Attitudes of low positive affect are associated with depression.

Depressive symptoms of 3,431 adolescents (ages 13–15 years) in Norway were investigated by Fandrem, San, and Roland (2009). They found that immigrant adolescents in Norway were more subject to depression than natives. Immigrants apparently suffer more from being deprived than natives and seek social services less. Female adolescents in Norway suffer greater depression than male adolescents. The authors reason that girls internalize their psychological problems while boys externalize them, thereby the difference. However, in this study, immigrant boys suffer greater depression than immigrant girls. The rural–urban differences are interesting. Previous studies have revealed scant difference between the two environments. This was the case – little difference between rural and urban – for adolescent girls, but not for boys. For boys, especially immigrants, depressive symptoms were more prevalent in urban environments than rural. The social work services available in urban areas apparently were not sought by immigrant boys in cities, whereas they were used by girls. Other studies have shown social support to be important in facilitating acculturation. Family support also makes a difference when depressive symptoms appear. The items used to measure depression in this study are interesting. They asked about the following depressive symptoms: blaming yourself for things; feeling everything is hard going; feeling unhappy, sad, or depressed; feeling hopeless about the future; worrying or stewing about things; difficulty in falling asleep or staying asleep.

Chronic stress is said to decrease longevity, induce other medical disabilities, and mar social relations. Specialists have cautioned patients with stress to take exercise to reduce anxiety and stress, to talk over stressful problems with friends, to interrupt the workday by relaxing in short breaks from work, and to find ways to maintain peace of mind. Advice such as this is designed to make life less complicated and stressful, and enhance the QOL.

Cognitive therapy and medication, both, come to the aid of depression and other mental disorders. Cognitive psychotherapy often is effective in mild cases. It involves four to ten visits to a psychiatrist. The procedure is to replace negative thoughts with a more positive, optimistic outlook. Other psychological techniques are applied, depending upon the patient's condition. Medical treatment has advanced notably during the past decade. Prozac is widely used. It affects the serotonin, endorphins, and dopamine of the brain. Prozac is not effective treatment for everyone, and for some, it has disagreeable side effects. The fact is that all drugs are toxic and all have side effects of one kind or another. However, experiments are going forward with other medications to treat mental conditions.

Psilocybin has been tried on volunteers with obsessive–compulsive disorder. Drugs are being tested to relieve posttraumatic stress disorder. The ayahuasca tea now is used in religious rituals in New Mexico, for its hallucinogenic effect (Marsa, 2008). The objective of such treatment is to return the sufferer to normality, so that a satisfying QOL may be enjoyed. We may expect medical science in the future to discover effective treatments for such mental conditions as these.

A survey of 4,849 subjects in 10 European countries and Israel found social support to be associated with better mental health. However, the effect of education on mental health varied among countries (Schmidt & Power, 2006).

One's mental condition, also, may be influenced through affiliation with a religious body. A study comparing coping practices of Christians, Muslims, Jews, and several other faiths showed that religious coping benefits mental health. In this study, coping with mental distress through prayer, listening to religious radio, using amulets, talking to God, and having a trusting relationship with God led to change in emotional states (Bhui, King, Dein, & O'Connor, 2008). Coping thus benefits mental health.

Stress

Uncertainties resulting from changes in oppressive social systems give rise to personal stress. Stress comes from anxiety about one's future, unsatisfactory interpersonal relationships, and inability to cope with annoying impositions. The consequences are high blood pressure, seeking release through alcohol or drugs, ulcers, depression, and other debilitating conditions. Stress hormones, adrenaline and cortisol, flow into the bloodstream. Blood sugar rises. Over time, repetition of this reaction affects the endocrine system. Havoc results. Colds and sniffles likely follow. The grinding of teeth, tension of muscles, and a fast heartbeat give signs of trouble ahead. But it need not destroy one's QOL. Seek release through laughing, crying, or shouting. Blow it out. Exercise regularly. Find sympathetic relatives and friends for reinforcement of altruism. Avoid fast food and eat nutritious balanced meals. Avoid overeating. Get into activities you enjoy, such as games, dancing, visiting, outdoor work like gardening, or working with wood. Recall the past difficulties that you have overcome. Try yoga, tai chi, meditation, or other means of focusing your attention. Breathe deeply and regularly. Finally, take steps to remedy whatever aspects of your situation for the better. Life will be better and your QOL will maintain itself.

Overweight, Obesity

An increasing segment of the population is overweight. Excess weight elevates the risk of morbidity and mortality through risk of heart disease, diabetes, some cancers, hypertension, arthritis, problems of weight on the bones, stroke, liver and gall-bladder diseases, and accidents. Extra weight is associated with several cancers, including colon, prostate, kidney, and breast. The obese are said to suffer sleep apnea. Persons gaining as little as two pounds in weight are said to increase their arthritis risk by 9–13% (Kauer & Rubman, 2007).

Obese younger persons are subject to high cholesterol, hypertension, and diabetes (US Department of Health and Human Services, 2005). The percent of obese and overweight adults, 20–74 years, began increasing around 1980 and by 1999–2002, it had reached 31%. At the same time, overweight children 6–11 years of age reached 15.8% and those 12–19 years reached 16%. A recent (2008) study from the CDC found 25.6% of the US adult population obese. The southern states, stretching from Texas to North Carolina, were more obese than the rest of the nation. The World Health Organization (WHO) estimates that worldwide, over 22 million children under age 5 years are overweight. More than 10% of children in developed countries pass as overweight, but overweight children also are increasing in developing countries, such as Argentina, Egypt, and South Africa (Ratzan et al., 2000).

The Centers for Disease Control and Prevention estimates that 80% of the 9 million adolescents who are currently overweight, when they grow up, will be obese adults. An article in the *New England Journal of Medicine* (2007) estimated that up to 37% of males and 44% of female adolescents in 2000 will be obese when they reach 35 years of age. In 2035, there should be 10,000 more cases of heart disease. This prospect will result in higher rates of mortality for these cohorts.

The poor are more obese and overweight than the non-poor, and females more so than males. Contributing to the problem are diets with excessive fat and sugar, low levels of exercise, sedentary lifestyles, and genetic influences. Solutions to the problem include changing lifestyle to more activity and exercise, reduction in consumption of fat, and improvement in nutrition in the diet. Promoting these objectives in order to improve the QOL is a public health problem of major proportions, involving schools, community agencies, and organizations.

Dr. Joel Fuhrman has developed a health equation, the ratio of nutrients to calories, and shows that per 100 calories, vegetables provide more nutrients than meat. His dietary program includes green vegetables, fresh fruit, beans and legumes, flaxseed, and one ounce of nuts, and limits or excludes starchy food and animal and dairy products (Fuhrman, 1999).

A recent study of 168 obese women who were awaiting bariatric surgery found obesity associated with poor QOL and poorer general health. They reported binge eating, continuous nibbling, and night eating. However, their sweet-fat food craving was not different from cravings of non-obese women (Silva et al., 2008).

Arthritis often accompanies obesity. A US study from the National Health Interview Survey found that persons with self-reported arthritis were 39.2% less than optimum on a Health-Related QOL scale. The study used 1986–1988 and 1994 survey data with 423,400 cases (Anderson, Kaplan, & Smith, 2004). In other studies, weight loss is advised for patients with the pain of arthritis. The literature abounds with advice for reducing pain and various nutritional strategies, such as fish oil (with omega-3), for reducing inflammation.

Regarding overweight and obesity, recent studies by Professor Kenneth Ferraro of Purdue University have found a relationship between religious affiliation and obesity. Baptists, he reports, are 30% obese, Catholics 17%, and the non-Christian religious followers, such as the Jews, Muslims, Hindus, and Buddhists, are only 1% obese (Salmon, 2007). Some religious groups have cited doctrinal support for maintaining a slender figure and have organized "faith-based" diet clubs. One Virginia Baptist pastor is said to have lost 70 pounds and from the pulpit advocated weight reduction as "your body is for the glorification of God."

The body mass index (BMI) reflects obesity when the weight divided by the square of the height exceeds 25. Studies have found the BMI related to a number of factors, including education, age, physical activity, income, and gender. A study of 700 Dutch citizens (Cornelisse-Vermaat, Judith, Antonides, Van Ophem, & Van Den Brink, 2006) found the BMI indirectly related negatively to happiness via perceived health. Being married was positively associated with health, as reported by the respondents. A combination of factors making for a regular lifestyle supports better perceived health and a lower BMI. While the authors warn that the results of their study may not generalize to persons in other cultures, they conclude that reducing the BMI will lead to better perceived health and greater happiness.

Rewarding fat loss has become a fad. Some business enterprises offer bonuses for fat reduction of employees. The idea is that it will improve health and reduce absenteeism. Manchester, England, rewards exercise and fat reduction by points, which, when accumulated, may be traded for purchase of athletic equipment or training sessions with athletes. Points are awarded by such healthy activities as the purchase of fruits and vegetables, swimming in a community pool, attending a medical screening, or working out with a personal trainer. The idea is to help people make healthier choices.

Advice abounds on how to lose weight. First steps include eating fruits and vegetables, grains and the like, instead of fat-laden foods such as meat and dairy products. Four ounces of fish once or twice a week is suggested for omega-3. Next in losing weight is activity: vigorous physical activity 30 min to 1 h daily. Walk, walk, walk, or bicycle, or ride horseback, but easiest and cheapest is walking. Do not avoid breakfast, as it helps to reduce daily calorie consumption. Aim for slow long-term reduction rather than quick off (and return) of fat. Checking weight weekly is advised. If a pound is gained, work immediately to lose it. Maintain whatever weight loss has been achieved. It is more important to lose regularly and slowly rather than rapidly. "Small changes drive success." The consequence will be an improved QOL and more attractive appearance.

Prevention

One approach to reducing the cost of medical care lies in preventing illness. Steps can be taken to reduce the probability of illness by changing lifestyle habits and practices. Stop smoking cigarettes. Reduce or eliminate alcohol consumption. Bring weight down to an acceptable body mass index (BMI). Exercise daily. Change diet to low fat, low protein, high fiber, vegetables, fruits, and grains. For many, these preventive steps would require a change in lifestyle, habits, and routines. But what are the consequences? Fewer trips to the doctor, greater vigor, and better health.

There also are medical steps to prevent illness. Take vaccine shots for the next round of influenza, diphtheria, measles, mumps, small pox, chicken pox, diphtheria, and other diseases, as medical science develops them. The increased amount of international travel has resulted in greater transmission of viruses from animals and from tropical countries. Public health officials must inspect, quarantine, and take other necessary steps to prevent international transmission. Medical science, also, can monitor the composition of the blood, identifying excessive cholesterol, potassium, blood sugar, and other elements that may be corrected by diet and medication before illness conditions result. Much can be done to prevent the development of illness.

Not all of the medical establishment is trained and equipped to provide prevention services. Rather, they are trained to identify illness conditions and treat them. But this is changing. Most recently, the Cleveland Clinic in Ohio has established a *Lifestyle 180* program. Its prevention program includes weight loss, stress reduction, high blood pressure reduction, dietary caution, exercise, cooking practices, and other wellness actions. Healthy behavior is rewarded, with cash if necessary.

In 1985, a program at the Cleveland Clinic began that showed the need for prevention. A surgeon, Dr. C.B Esselstyn, Jr., MD (2007), hit upon a dietary treatment for heart disease. The cardiologists at the Clinic assigned 24 patients with advanced coronary artery disease to Dr. Esselstyn's experiment in nutrition. They were patients whom the physicians could no longer benefit, patients to be sent home to the rocking chair. Dr. Esselstyn explained the dietary program to them. It consisted of plant-based foods devoid of animal protein or fat. The objective was to reduce cholesterol to 150 mg/dL or lower. At this level, plaque would no longer accumulate in the arteries. Six declined to enter his program and were returned to standard care. The remainder began a routine of plant-based food in their diet. They met with the doctor every 2 weeks to review their food intake. They were assigned medication to reduce cholesterol. Dr. Esselstyn followed them for 12 years, the longest such medical study. Of those following the diet, only one died, and one who did not comply fully required by-pass surgery. The remainder after 12 years experienced no coronary events. The six who did not enter the program experienced worsening heart disease. Altogether, after 12 years, they experienced 13 episodes, one being a mortality. The experiment was a notable success. "Among the fully compliant patients, during the 12-year study, there was not one further clinical episode of worsening coronary artery disease after they committed themselves to keeping cholesterol within the safe range" (p. 55). The experiment is described, along with the diet, in the book *Prevent and Reverse Heart Disease* (2007, Penguin). It showed that the progress of coronary heart disease could be reversed through diet. A comparable program under Dr. Dean Ormish has shown similar results.

Alcoholism

One source of ill-health is alcoholism. It also interferes with or disrupts attainment of Mastery, Intellectual Autonomy, Social Acceptance, and other domains of the QOL. Consequently, the means for changing to a nonalcoholic lifestyle becomes important for attaining good health. Twenty million Americans are thought to suffer alcohol abuse, yet only 2 million are engaged in a treatment program.

Use of alcohol is indeed a risk factor, causing disability and illness that can be corrected. In 2001, 48.3% of persons 12 years of age and over used alcohol during the past month. One-fifth of the population reported "binge" use of the drug. In 2005, three-quarters of high school seniors reported using alcohol. Alcohol consumption is most prevalent among young adults, 18–24 years of age (National Center for Health Statistics, 2003; Kashner, 2007).

Over a 2-year period, 1996–1998, a mean of 9.6 alcohol-related deaths per 100,000 adults 18 years and older in Florida counties were reported. This figure, 9.6 per 100,000 compares with 4.3 drug-related deaths. However, arrests for driving under the influence of alcohol were 786 per 100,000 for Florida counties in the same 2-year period. Hospital discharges for the treatment of alcohol abuse disorders and for diseases and injuries attributable to alcohol abuse were 143/100,000 for Florida counties. During the same period, there were 2,103 highway crashes involving drivers under the influence of alcohol as determined by the investigating law enforcement officer (Solzenberg & associates, 2003). The study included other substance abuse in addition to alcohol for the 67 counties of Florida, and provides a social indicator approach to establishing the need for remedial services in the counties.

In 1937, Harvard scholars initiated a longitudinal study of 268 sophomores and continued to collect responses from them for 72 years. The sample represents a select set of educationally elite and professionally promising men. This remarkable study design enables inferences of the pressures and habits that lead to alcoholism. By age 50, one third of the men met the investigators' criteria of mental illness. Those who exercised during college years were in better mental health in later life than was their physical condition. Those diagnosed with depression at age 50 were either deceased or critically ill by age 63. World War II had its impact on their lives. Those who survived heavy combat developed more chronic physical illness and died sooner than those who saw no combat. Dr. George Vallant, a psychiatrist, was so impressed by the impact of alcohol on the men that he published *The Natural History of Alcoholism*, based upon the cohort data. He magnifies the importance of social relationships in successful aging. Successful aging, he says, hinges upon, not intelligence nor social status, but upon "social aptitude." Nearly all men who were thriving at age 65, when younger, had been close to their sibs. The case studies show the effect of the gradual increase in alcohol consumption that leads eventually to alcoholism. They also show a corresponding deterioration in marital and social relationships (Shenk, 2009).

Psychiatric treatment, medical attention, religious conversion, social group influence, and other means enable the alcoholic to assume a sober lifestyle. The Alcoholics Anonymous program has helped many, but statistical proof of effectiveness is difficult to acquire. It works through local organizations of AA groups and through books and inspirational, religious literature. The alcoholic assembles with other now-sober former alcoholics to hear testimonies of recovery, thus demonstrating that a life without alcohol is possible and enjoyable. The alcoholic is urged by former alcoholics to assume sobriety through following a 12-step program. It involves encouragement from former alcoholics, spiritual and other appeals, as follows:

1. We admitted we were powerless over alcohol – that our lives had become unmanageable.
2. Came to believe that a Power greater than ourselves could restore us to sanity.
3. Made a decision to turn our will and our lives over to the care of God, *as we understood Him.*

4. Made a searching and fearless moral inventory of ourselves.
5. Admitted to God, to ourselves, and to another human being the exact nature of our wrongs.
6. Were entirely ready to have God remove all these defects of character.
7. Humbly asked Him to remove our shortcomings.
8. Made a list of all persons we had harmed, and became willing to make amends to them all.
9. Made direct amends to such people wherever possible, except when to do so would injure them or others.
10. Continued to take personal inventory and when we were wrong promptly admitted it.
11. Sought through prayer and meditation to improve our conscious contact with God, *as we understood Him*, praying only for knowledge of His will for us and the power to carry that out.
12. Having had a spiritual awakening as the result of these steps, we tried to carry this message to alcoholics, and to practice these principles in all our affairs.

The above are quoted from the Al-Anon literature (Al-Anon, 1995). The spiritual aspects of the program are evident in the 12 steps, but the social aspects, involving interaction with reformed alcoholics, stand as a cornerstone of the program. The steps are said to be an expansion of the Oxford Group program. The Oxford Group principles are the following: (1) To seek Divine Guidance in all aspects of life. (2) To humble myself to God and surrender completely to Him. (3) To acknowledge any offences against others. (4) To make restitution to those sinned against. (4) To promote the group to the public in an evangelical manner. Because of these principles, some critics describe AA as a religious cult (Mohr, 2009). Some courts assign alcoholics to AA for "treatment." Some consider this action illegal and unconstitutional. Better, the critics say, would be treatment by Food and Drug Administration approved medications, such as Topamax, Campral, and Vivitrol, the latter blocking the alcohol effect in the brain (Mohr, 2009).

Daily or weekly Alcoholics Anonymous meetings follow a standard routine of reading the purposes of the meeting and repeating the 12 steps.

When presenting a testimonial, the speaker announces his/her first name, never more, and describes experience with alcohol, the pitfalls and degradation into which he/she had fallen, and comments upon the joys of new life without liquor.

An alcoholic attempting to reform may feel tempted, and, in desperation, telephone or call upon a member of AA for help and support. AA members always stand ready to aid persons calling for help, service to recovering alcoholics being part of the 12th step. The AA organization publishes inspirational and self-help books. They provide instruction and inspiration for families and friends of alcoholics.

Al-Anon in its meetings follows similar steps, the emphasis here being to help members of the alcoholic's family or loved ones adjust to the problems of living with an alcoholic. Meetings begin with a "Serenity Prayer" followed by recitation of a welcome to newcomers and statement of purpose of the organization. The 12 steps are reviewed. Members voluntarily give anonymous testimonials, expressing problems of dealing with alcoholic members of the family or of friends. The meetings usually maintained a relaxed atmosphere with laughter. Meetings end, as do AA meetings, with a prayer.

A combination of pharmaceutical and social treatment appears to be the most effective approach to eliminating dependence upon alcohol. Several medical treatments have been approved by the US Food and Drug Administration.

> *Disulfiram* (Antabuse) in the 1990s brought home to alcoholics the nausea of consuming it. The drug interferes with the metabolism of alcohol. By taking 250–500 mg daily, an alcoholic will experience violent nausea upon ingesting alcohol. This severe negative reaction to alcohol reduces desire and is a powerful deterrent to drinking.
>
> *Naltrexone* (ReVia) taken daily in 50 mg doses is considered a short-term treatment for alcoholism. It is considered effective when used in conjunction with socio-psychological counseling. In the brain, it blocks receptors of natural painkillers, called opioids. These create the pleasurable feeling associated with drinking alcohol.
>
> *Topiramate* has been approved for treatment of epilepsy, cocaine addiction, and alcoholism.
>
> *Baclofen* is for muscle tightness, cramping and spasms, and for alcoholism.
>
> *Ondansetron* treats nausea and vomiting and has been approved for alcoholism.
>
> *Nalmefene*, approved in 1994 for alcoholism, is now being considered as a treatment for opiate addiction.
>
> *Buprenorphine* (trade name Suboxone and Subutex) became available in 2003 to treat heroin, painkiller, and opiate addictions, and alcoholism. It can be prescribed by physicians in private practice.

Total abstinence should be the objective of treatment programs for alcoholics.

In addition to Alcoholics Anonymous, other groups are concerned with the problem. The University of Pennsylvania has developed a medical model for treatment, based upon a 20-year history of clinical studies. The American Council on Alcoholism provides information on treatment options and refers alcoholics for treatment. The National Clearinghouse on Alcohol and Drug Information provides written material on alcohol and drug-related subjects. A National Council on Alcoholism and Drug Dependence Helpline provides an advisory and referral service. These agencies have websites where additional information is available. There are many books describing successful treatment, with encouraging stories for alcoholics.

Cigarettes

Cigarette smoking is associated with an increased risk of heart disease, stroke, lung cancer, and chronic lung disease, according to the Centers for Disease Control and Prevention. Since the Federal program against it began, success in reducing smoking has been notable. Since 1965, the percent of men who smoke cigarettes has declined from 51.2 to 24.7% in 2001. Similarly, women smokers have declined from 33.7 to 20.8%. Smoking by youth has posed a problem. The smoking rate among high school students reached a peak in 1995 of nearly 35%, but it since has declined to 28.5% in 2001. The number of years of schooling is associated with smoking. Those with less than high school graduation are three times more likely to smoke than college graduates. Smoking also varies for ethnic groups and by region.

Over the past 15 years, the percent smoking has declined at about 0.4% per year, being 21% in 2006. In 2001, among persons 25 years and over, males (23.9%) were more frequent smokers than females.

The US Surgeon General began concerted attacks against smoking in 1964. His landmark report cited some 7,000 studies linking smoking to disease. Some 434,000 deaths annually are attributed to tobacco use. Cigarette smoking causes 21% of heart disease deaths, 87% of lung cancer deaths, and 82% of chronic obstructive pulmonary disease.

The medical model was initially adopted, in which individual smokers were advised to quit by their physician. It was not effective. The program shifted to an environmental approach that advocated increases in taxes on cigarettes, restricting smoking in public places, and other measures. The Federal Cigarette Labeling and Advertising Act of 1965 and the Public Health Cigarette Smoking Act of 1969 required cigarette packages to include a warning of injury to health from cigarette use. Radio and TV broadcasting of cigarette advertising was banned. State legislatures joined the fight in 1985. After 1988, they passed 1,239 laws addressing tobacco use. These measures were effective in reducing the practice. Lester F. Ward, around the turn of the twentieth century, used the term "telesis" to designate efforts to institute change through legislative initiatives. Telesis has been most effective in reducing the use of tobacco.

A recent study (Kaplan, Robert, Anderson, & Kaplan, 2006) assembled data from the National Health Interview Survey on a sample of people ages 18–70 and followed them through death records for 6 years. Tobacco use was found to decrease health-related QOL and decrease life expectancy. Results of the study provide support for investment in preventing the use of tobacco, particularly among young adults. "The tobacco prevention programs may produce a full 5 years of life for those individuals prevented from smoking by age 20" (p. 60). The study reported that increases in taxes on tobacco added quality years of life. It reports on the *Smoking Cessation Clinical Practice Guidelines* developed by the Agency for Health Care Policy and Research. The report estimates the cost/benefit of various cease-smoking protocols.

Cigarette smoking by mentally ill persons also is a problem. About half the cigarettes sold in the United States are purchased by the mentally ill. Well-meaning persons reason that stopping smoking should not be forced upon the mentally ill, owing to their disabilities. However, now about half of the hospitals for the mentally ill are smoke free.

Nine recent studies of second-hand smoke reveal that heart attacks have decreased after smoking was banned from workplaces. Authorities assert that smoke-free environments are an effective means of reducing heart and cancer incidence. Second-hand smoke is recognized as a cause of lung cancer. Statistics assembled by the Center for Disease Control and Prevention estimate that 46,000 die annually, with 3,000 lung cancer deaths among nonsmokers. Evidence of the effectiveness of banning smoking in public places resulted in a reduction in heart attacks from 257/100,000 to 152/100,000 over 3 years. The area studied was Pueblo County, the city of Pueblo, and El Paso County, Colorado.

To halt worldwide tobacco consumption and exposure to cigarette smoke, a Framework Convention on Tobacco Control was organized in 2003 with the support of the World Health Organization. The treaty has been ratified by 161 countries. Increasing taxes on the sale of tobacco products is one "telic" step governments may take in an effort to reduce consumption. Another is advertising the danger to health of tobacco consumption. Restricting smoking in public places, allowing it only outdoors and in designated rooms has become the means of reducing exposure to second-hand smoke. Nonsmokers enjoy a better QOL and longer life expectancy.

Exercise

The single most beneficial health activity is walking regularly. According to several studies, rapid walking only 30 min for 6 days a week reduces the risk of stroke, reduces blood pressure, decreases the probability of heart attack, lowers the risk of vascular dementia and trims the waistline. It does not cost anything. Walk for better health. Similarly, beneficial are bicycle or horseback riding, swimming, and jogging.

Unless we use them as we age, our muscles become soft and smaller. To prevent this, we need to lift weights or work out on machines that offer resistance. Twenty to thirty minutes several, say three, times a week strengthening the major muscle groups will keep the body strong. Those not in top form should begin with small weights, perhaps two pounds, and repeat the motion until fatigued, 10 or 12 times. Then, the weight should be gradually increased, as well as the number of repetitions. Muscles should be allowed to relax and restore before the next work-out.

Oxygen is used throughout the body, the brain, the heart, the lungs, and the muscles. In addition to rapid walking, aerobic exercise, more vigorous, brings on perspiration and a flushed face. It will help to ward off many conditions, including high blood pressure, overweight, diabetes, stroke, and some cancers. Thirty minutes to one hour several times a week are sufficient to keep a person in top form. It helps to exercise with a partner. Joining a group with a leader makes it easier to make the most of it, and working with others helps to motivate. Stress is reduced and mental health problems modified by sustained 20-min physical activity, any kind – gardening, walking, engaging in sports, etc. – according to a study published in the *British Journal of Sports Medicine*. In engaging in an exercise program for health, one will improve one's balance by shifting from one leg to the other. Gaining flexibility through stretching, as with yoga, improves core stability and gives better control of movements. Both yoga and tai chi emphasize balance and muscle tone. Regularly engaged, these exercises keep a person feeling in charge and lead to a better QOL.

Nutrition

Rather frequently, medical research reports benefits to health of specific vitamins. Many medical professionals recommend daily ingestion of a multiple vitamin.

Food provides sufficient vitamins if the diet follows the recommended balance of fruits, vegetables, grains, and fibers. Nutritionists recommend eating meats only occasionally, because eating excessive fats and protein are associated with cancer and other malignancies.

Dr. Joel Fuhrman, MD, recommends lowering LDL cholesterol the natural way, through eating vegetables, fruits, nuts, and grains, and avoiding meats and dairy products. His recommendations include losing weight (if it is high), boosting the immune function, lowering high blood pressure, preventing autoimmune diseases, and maintaining youthful vigor through exercise and rest (Fuhrman, 2004).

Vitamin D has been found to facilitate the absorption of calcium for the bones. It will help reduce osteoporosis, which is a growing menace among older Americans. It is estimated that 12 million people in the United States suffer from osteoporosis, and another 40 million have low bone mass as they age. The body manufactures vitamin D when exposed to the sun, but often people receive insufficient exposure to sunlight. In a normal diet, 10–15% of the calcium in the diet is absorbed. With vitamin D, absorption is increased to 30–50% of calcium. The US Food and Drug Administration approved in 2003 the addition of vitamin D to calcium-fortified juices. These results are chiefly from the Boston University Medical School's Bone Health Research Laboratory.

The Archives of Internal Medicine published a study that quoted Rashni Sinaha of the National Cancer Institute that found that men and women who ate a quarter pound of hamburger daily had a higher risk of dying of heart disease and cancer than those who ate less than one ounce of red meat daily. The study included 47,976 men and 23,276 women who died over a 10-year period, ranging in age from 50 to 71 years. Meat eaters were more likely to die during the 10-year period, even after other factors were accounted for, factors such as eating fruits and vegetables, smoking, exercise, and obesity. Bowel and lung cancer, also, have been linked with eating red and processed meats, according to the US National Cancer Institute. The result of these studies is that eating less or no red meat will improve longevity and health.

A comprehensive study of nutrition practices in China by T. Colin Campbell of Cornell University (2005), *The China Study*, found that the plant-based diet of rural Chinese prevented the acquisition of heart disease, cancer, and other diseases common to America. Animal fat appears to be the culprit. A country-by-country chart of fat intake and breast cancer mortality shows a high correlation, in the 0.90s. Dietary fat is low in such countries as Thailand, Japan, Mexico, and El Salvador, where the age-adjusted death rate is near zero, to high-fat countries, such as the Netherlands, UK, Denmark, Canada, and New Zealand, where the breast cancer mortality is in the range of 25 per 100,000 females.

Sixty-five counties across China were selected for study, which included 6,500 individuals. The sample had consumed the same diet and had lived in the same place all their lives. Compared to the United States, the China sample consumed 33% more calories, 60% less fat, 175% more dietary fiber, and 30% less total protein. The animal protein consumed by the Chinese amounted to only 0.8% of calories, while in the United States, it amounted to 11% of calories. These estimates are for a standardized 143 pound person. The comparison led to the conclusion that "a diet high in animal-based protein can have unfavorable health consequences " (p. 277). They also led to eight principles of nutrition and health, set forth, which are as follows:

1. "Nutrition represents the combined activities of countless food substances. The whole is greater than the sum of the parts." By this, Campbell means that plant-based foods include a wide variety of nutrients that the body uses to vitalize its cells.
2. "Vitamin supplements are not a panacea for good health."
3. "There are virtually no nutrients in animal-based foods that are not better provided by plants." The nutritional value of the plant-based diet far exceeds that of the animal, according to a chart that compares the two, based upon 500 calories of energy and approximately equal grams of protein (33–34 g).
4. "Genes do not determine disease on their own. Genes function only by being activated, or expressed, and nutrition plays a critical role in determining which genes, good and bad are expressed."
5. "Nutrition can substantially control the adverse effects of noxious chemicals."
6. "The same nutrition that prevents disease in its early stages (before diagnosis) can also halt or reverse disease in its later stages (after diagnosis)."
7. "Nutrition that is truly beneficial for one chronic disease will support health across the board." The implication of this principle is that one can maximize health across the board by one simple diet: plant-based foods.
8. "Good nutrition creates health in all areas of our existence. All parts are interconnected." In addition to nutrition's impact on health, eating plant-based foods also benefits the environment. Plant foods require less water to cultivate than do animal foods with the same calorie structure, less land, fewer resources, less pollution, and no suffering of farm animals. Good nutrition based upon plants promises to sustain the planet in many ways.

These eight principles, formulated by T. Colin Campbell in *The China Study*, come out of a lifetime of study of nutritional biochemistry as well as the epidemiological study of China.

Health Summary

More healthy days are associated with better QOL.

Health is impacted by cultural traditions affecting nutrition and lifestyle.

Life expectancy is usually longer in richer countries.

Educating women reduces child mortality.

The better educated are healthier than the less educated.

Better health may come from walking, aerobics, yoga and tai chi, and other exercises.

In future, technology promises to improve health and bodily functioning.

Western medicine is being modified by alternative treatments such as acupuncture, meditation, herbs, touching, etc.

Stress hampers good health. Exercise helps. Mental illness distresses a growing segment of people. Drugs and cognitive therapy can be applied.

Obesity, a health detriment, may be reduced by exercise and a diet of vegetables, fruits, grains, etc.

Alcoholism can be overcome through AA and medication.

Cigarette smoking is declining but still poses a threat worldwide. Legislative action on the conditions of smoking has reduced the practice.

Chapter 11
Toward the Good Life in a Good Society

> A general definition of civilization:
> A civilized society is exhibiting the
> five qualities of Truth, Beauty,
> Adventure, Art, Peace.
> *–Alfred North Whitehead, Adventures in Ideas, Chap. 19*

> One should get rid of a selfish mind and replace it with a mind that is earnest to help others. An act to make another happy inspires the other to make still another happy, and so happiness is born from such an act.
> *–Purification of the Mind, Chapter 1, The Way of Purification, in The Teaching of Buddha (1996)*

> A good society is a means to a good life for those who compose it; not something having a kind of excellence on its own account.
> *–Bertrand Russell, Authority and the Individual.*

The Good Society. The good life flourishes in the good society, with appropriate social structure, social psychology, values, and culture patterns. Finding the good society will yield keys to the good life.

Proposition 11. The social structure and social psychology of the good society may be found by identifying situations where good QOL of the people predominates. The good society will involve norms and values, social quality, structural relationships, and other such qualities of societies.

Values

A normative basis is required for a good society, according to discussions in 2000 at Frankfurt, Germany, at a meeting of the German Sociological Congress. Basic consensus on goals of society is needed in development of the good society. All domains of QOL serve as criteria for what should be achieved in order to have a good society.

A good society creates conditions for happiness of its members. At the Congress, sustainability and cohesion were advanced as requirements for the good society. It considered that the diverse sectors of society should be integrated. The family and intergenerational relations came into discussion. Is the welfare state necessary for the good society? Both sides of the issue were presented. East Germans sided with

A.L. Ferriss, *Approaches to Improving the Quality of Life*, Social Indicators Research Series 42, DOI 10.1007/978-90-481-9148-2_11, © Springer Science+Business Media B.V. 2010 the concepts of the West, rather than supporting the former East German system. Ideals for the good society included freedom, equality, and solidarity. The group was reminded that ambivalence is a basic feature of all societies (Glatzer, 2001) (see also Chapter 8).

Social Quality

Social quality is defined as "the extent to which citizens are able to participate in the social and economic life of their communities under conditions which enhance their well-being and individual potential" (attributed to W.L. Beck and others in the document *The Social Quality of Europe*). There are four major concepts of the notion of social quality: socioeconomic security, social inclusion, social cohesion, and empowerment. The chapter outlines the conceptual orientation of the social quality program (Berman & Philips, 2000) (see Chapter 9).

The four basic concepts may be better understood by the following from Burman and Phillips (2000):

Socio-economic security/insecurity refers to the way the essential needs of citizens with respect to their daily existence are addressed by the different systems and structures responsible for welfare provisions. An acceptable minimum of social–economic security provides protection against poverty, unemployment, ill-health and other forms of material deprivation.

Social inclusion/exclusion is connected with the principles of equality and equity and the structural causes of their existence. The goal is a basic level of inclusion with help of supportive infrastructures, labour conditions and collective goods in such a way that those mechanisms causing exclusion will be prevented or minimized. This element focuses attention on the structural causes of exclusion.

Social cohesion/anomie concerns the processes which create, defend or abolish social networks and the social infrastructures underpinning the networks. An adequate level of social cohesion is one which enables citizens to exist as real human subjects, as social beings. On the other hand, anomie is fostered by regional disparities, the suppression of minorities, unequal access to public goods and services and an unequal sharing of economic burdens.

Empowerment/disempowerment is the realization of human competencies and capabilities in order to fully participate in the social, economic, political and cultural processes. It primarily concerns enabling people as citizens, to develop their full potential.

Happiness

Bengt Brulde has edited an issue devoted to the relation of happiness to the good life (Brulde, 2007). In it, five scholars explore happiness as aspects of the good life. How necessary is happiness for one's quality of life? Arguments are advanced that there is more to life than mere happiness. One's evaluation of a life situation as good becomes an important aspect of one's conception of happiness, whether cognitive or affective. A "pure happiness theory" is rejected. One must assess life realistically. Such an assessment of one's life situation leads to a more solid belief in one's happiness. This is done by taking into account the major life domains that influence well-being. It remains that happiness is a key component of the good life. To be rational about one's situation and to face life with freedom are necessary ingredients of happiness and the good life. Other elements make up the good life: health, relationships, etc. The condition of happiness differs between individuals: what makes one person happy may not do the same for another.

Several national indices involving happiness have been proposed. A Happy Planet Index is available from the internet (www.happyplanetindex.org). It combines a nation's average happiness index with life expectancy. Yew-Kang Ng (2008) has modified it to incorporate a measure of environmental toxins, calling it ERHNI, Environmentally Responsible Happy Nation Index. He calculated it for 142 nations. With a world average of 4.705, African nations stand at −0.477, Middle East and Central Asia 2.982, Asia Pacific 5.158, Latin America and Caribbean 10.104, North America 8.378, Western Europe 11.883, and Central and Eastern Europe −0.691. Western Europe achieved the highest QOL, according to the index. These numbers are weighted averages, reflecting the population dimension. Switzerland heads the list with 22.789, followed, as might be expected, by Denmark with 19.339 and Sweden with 18.534.

One would expect war-torn nations to score low on the ERHNI. Of seven nations where the UN has peacekeeping missions, five have negative indexes, Sudan, for example, −8.033. By this criterion, the index appears sensitive to reality. Bhutan, the country that has officially declared the QOL and happiness as the criteria for progress, is not rated, probably for absence of data. Such indicators as these provide a substitute for GDP and GNP, which have been used to assess national well-being. International comparisons enable countries to evaluate their socioeconomic and political structure with the view to improving happiness and well-being. The road to happiness is further outlined in Chapter 4.

Peace

The major deterrent worldwide to the good life is international armed conflict. The United Nations Security Council, with 15 members, has responsibility and oversight for maintaining peace. Serving the interests of the common man and listening to the common voice may be the best ways to dampen threats of conflict (see Chapter 1).

Security

Regional political assemblies of states are brought together for various purposes, some chiefly economic, some for security, some for communication and exchange of information. States that communicate can reduce tensions and maintain a comity among nations. The Group of Eight includes the economically most powerful countries. Other assemblies and the size of their membership are as follows: African Union, 23 members; Asia-Pacific Economic Cooperation, 22 members; Association of Southeast Asian Nations, 10 members; Caribbean Community and Common Market, 19 members and 6 associate members; The Commonwealth, 53 members; Commonwealth of Independent States, 12 members; European Free Trade Association, 4 members; European Union, 25 members plus 70 affiliates; International Criminal Police Organization, 186 members; League of Arab States, 22 members; North Atlantic Treaty Organization, 26 members; Organization of American States, 39 members; Organization for Economic Cooperation and Development, 30 members; Organization of Petroleum Exporting Countries, 11 members; and Organization for Security and Cooperation in Europe, 56 members. In settling disputes between nations, these organizations reduce tension. Their actions give hope for a more harmonious world (see Chapter 1).

Plagues and Pandemics

Malaria, tuberculosis, HIV/AIDS, and other infections cause much suffering and death. Viruses arise out of the environment. About one-third of deaths worldwide are caused by parasitic and infectious diseases. They are public health problems of great moment. Each cause must be addressed according to its distinctive attributes, such as mosquito nets against malaria, vaccines against viruses, following the latest scientific developments. Condoms provide protection from HIV/AIDS, but they are not always used. Another method of protection, the use of microbicides in women, is being developed for use against HIV infection (see Chapter 10).

Religion

Religious organizations have brought peace and harmony, comfort, and solace to many. The social bonds of members and the sociability of participation contribute to life satisfaction and the QOL. Conflict between religious groups because of different beliefs, historically, has caused widespread loss of life and depletion of the QOL. Religious leaders must seek to eliminate interfaith conflict and promote harmony. Until such time as spirituality and other benefits of transcendent thought prevail, differences in belief must be tolerated and respected. If religious bodies fail to bring this about, or do not modify unrealistic theological positions, the other benefits of religious participation will be lost. Some of these benefits are sociability, celebration of life's turning points, social support, peace of mind, and ethical conduct. This is discussed in Chapter 3.

Religious participation and membership benefit one's health. Studies show that these activities lead to better health, lower blood pressure, lower rates of some cancers, longer life, and other advantages. Knowing that friends and acquaintances are concerned over one's well-being enhances one's self-concept. It stimulates concern for others and reinforces healthy habits to the end that the QOL is improved.

The ethical principles espoused by Judeo-Christian thought provide the basis for the good life, according to Peter J. Gomes (2002). In the book of Micah 6, we are told what is good: "to do justice, to love kindness and to walk humbly with your God." To this Gomes add the Christian virtue to love God and love your neighbor as yourself. Gomes expands upon this theme of the ethical basis of the good life. In addition to the Golden Rule, "humility, modesty, honesty, integrity, fidelity, fortitude, and courage" are virtues leading to the good life. Gomes says we will be happy if we do virtuous things, as defined here. "(H)appiness is a consequence of goodness" (p. 210). He quotes St. Thomas Aquinas as identifying the qualities that lead to the Christian life as "prudence, justice, temperance and fortitude."

Saint Paul is quoted as identifying the evils of the flesh. For the good life, these are to be avoided: "fornication, impurity, licentiousness, idolatry, sorcery, enmity, strife, jealousy, anger, selfishness, dissension, party spirit, envy, drunkenness, carousing and the like." At the other extreme, Paul admonishes "faith, hope and love, but the greatest of these is love." Following these precepts, Gomes expounds upon discipline, freedom, faith, hope, and love. These virtues, he says, lead to the good life (Gomes, 2002).

Buddhist philosophy sets forth an eightfold path to "enlightenment." The Noble Eightfold Path is deeply psychological and is the basis of the practice that forms the nexus of the spiritual and practical teachings, leading to the good life. The eight aspects are as follows:

"Right View means to thoroughly understand the Fourfold Truth, to believe in the law of cause and effect and not to be deceived by appearances and desires."

"Right Thought means the resolution not to cherish desires, not to be greedy, not to be angry, and not to do any harmful deed."

"Right Speech means the avoidance of lying words, idle words, abusive words, and double tongues."

"Right Behavior means not to destroy any life, not to steal, or not to commit adultery."

"Right Livelihood means to avoid any life that would bring shame."

"Right Effort means to try to do one's best diligently toward the right direction."

"Right Mindfulness means to maintain a pure and thoughtful mind."

"Right Concentration means to keep the mind right and tranquil for its concentration, seeking to realize the mind's pure essence."

The Fourfold Noble Truth, referred to above, consists of four causes of suffering: the Truth of Suffering, The Truth of the Cause of Suffering (which is intense desires of physical instincts), the Truth of the Cessation of the Cause of Suffering, and the Truth of the Noble Path to the Cessation of the Cause of Suffering (Kyokai, 1990).

Buddhist values, loving kindness, compassion, and joy, were combined in a scale by Kraus and Sears (2009). They found the scale strongly associated with other psychological dimensions: a cognitive and affective mindfulness scale (which taps attention, present focus, awareness, and acceptance aspects of mindfulness), and a positive and negative affect scale. While the Buddhist values scale is associated with positive and negatively associated with negative psychological moods, the scale is not posed against general QOL. However, the scale may find use in later studies that examine the relationship of religious values with the QOL.

Thus we have the Judeo-Christian path to the good life and the Buddhist concern with the psyche as the path to enlightenment. Devotion to the religious way of life would entail following the principles herewith set forth in order to attain the good life.

Demographic Growth

Population growth directly affects the QOL. Excessive growth because of high-fertility should be reduced through planned parenthood methods. Some religious groups oppose this for theological reasons. Countries below replacement levels, as are some parts of Europe, should promote fertility through state programs of tax reduction, relief of the pregnant female from work, and other such incentives. Population growth in sub-Saharan Africa is declining because of mortality from HIV/AIDS, especially in Botswana and Zimbabwe. However, sub-Saharan Africa's population will increase as a proportion of world population.

Population growth should be consistent with the needs of the economic system of the country so that unemployment is minimized, and also minimized is the impact of growth on the environment. Demographers anticipate a 2050 world population of around 9 billion. In low-fertility countries, the average age of the population will be older than today's. High-fertility countries will have a younger average age. Future population will be heavily concentrated in urban areas. Worldwide, a greater proportion will be living in Africa and a smaller proportion in North America and Europe. If this shift materializes, the QOL will be threatened by overpopulation and the adverse effects of climate change. This is a strong possibility.

The population expansion now being experienced and expected in the future is directly related to the overproduction of carbon dioxide and other toxic gases in the upper atmosphere. These gases cause climate change, global warming, and disappearance of glaciers. Thus, future population growth will cause further damage to the environment and deplete the QOL worldwide (see also Chapters 1 and 6). The ultimate goal is zero population growth.

Social and Individual Factors

Self-destruction

The causes of suicide are many, reviewed in Chapter 1. Extensive immigration has brought strangers into an unfamiliar culture, causing personal culture conflict and disorganization. Suicide results. One important preventive would be through social organization that ensured a close bond between the individual and a meaningful group that provides a reason for living.

Domestic Violence

The reduction of domestic violence should begin with emphasis upon familial love, advocated by P. A. Sorokin. When police intervene in family issues, they often augment rather than placate the situation. Conflict resolution is required, as discussed in Chapter 5. The practice of conflict resolution will reduce dissension in the family. Conflict resolution services should be provided by welfare and security organizations in each community. Otherwise, shelters for those in danger will temporarily reduce the violence but not remove the threat. Domestic harmony begins with consideration and love.

Mental Health

In the interest of a "flourishing" mental health, Keyes has pointed to a number of steps that lead to better QOL (Chapter 2). These include maintaining positive rather than negative attitudes, seeking satisfaction in life, contributing to the community, accepting others who may differ from one's self, understanding and accepting uniquely different traits, developing positive relations with others, finding ways to personal growth, and pursuing a purpose in life. While these do not exhaust the steps toward better mental health, if practiced, they would move one in the direction of a better QOL.

Physical Health

Given a body free of impairments, good nutrition, exercise, rest, and relaxation will lead to a good life, as described in Chapter 10. For good health, one should avoid ingesting toxins such as alcohol, tobacco, caffeine, and mind altering drugs.

Exercise, sauna, fasting, and sweating and excretion divest the body of these toxins.

Stress, depression, and other debilitating conditions may be reduced by exercise and other steps when they first appear.

Nutritious food will reduce the probability of many ailments: acne, appendicitis, atherosclerosis, allergies, angina, asthma, arthritis, constipation, colonic polyps, diabetes II, diverticulitis, esophagis, fibromyalgia, gallstones, gastritis, gout, headaches, hemorrhoids, high blood pressure, hypoglycemic symptoms, indigestion, irritable bowel syndrome, kidney stones, lumbar spine syndromes, muscular degeneration, musculoskeletal pain, osteoporosis, sexual dysfunction, stroke, uterine fibroids, and others (Fuhrman, 2003, p. 144). Nutritious food comes from a diet of fruits and vegetables, grains, and fiber (Chapter 10).

Socializing the Child

In the family, the child should be socialized in such a manner that develops self-esteem and self-control. The family, the neighborhood, the school, and the community each have a role in producing well-adjusted children, as discussed in Chapter 2. Wholesome development, free of stress, will arise from well-adjusted families with a satisfactory QOL.

Community and Neighborhood

In the neighborhood, one should participate in group activities, such as block parties, visiting one another's homes, assisting one's friends, and the like. These activities bolster one's self-concept and lead to social cohesion, as reviewed in Chapter 9. Neighborhood problems and crime was identified as a latent variable in a study of material*hardship* in the United States (Carle Bauman, & Short, 2009). The study assembled a large set of factors from the US Survey of Income and Program Participation, identified as consumer durables, resources available to meet needs, housing conditions, neighborhood problems and crime, and community services, identified by factor analysis. The study found that subjective evaluations related closely to the hardship factors.

A study by Baker and Palmer (2006) provides a model for relating participation in community recreation and other activities, but the small sample size ($n = 352$) (a selected sample of 1,100) representing 175,000 residents of a southwestern US community renders the results questionable. They found that community pride and community facilities (elements) were strong predictors of the QOL. Recreation participation showed a negative relation to QOL as also did length of residence. The authors' model, showing the interaction of community participation, pride, facilities (elements), and residency to the quality of life and satisfaction, may be considered in future studies, but the study lacks adequate sample responses for reliable results. We remain, then, with the hypothesis that QOL may be built by involvement in community activities, through recreation participation, adult education activities, outdoor leisure time, artistic endeavors, and related involvements.

Leisure Time

One should find expressive activities in one's leisure moments, such as arts and crafts, adventures such as hiking in the wilderness, fishing, and the like (see Chapter 2). This contrasts starkly with drinking beer while watching an athletic contest, which has no place in the good life. Making something with one's hands, a picture, a basket, a sled – anything – leads to essential and lasting satisfaction. The sensation of awe at Nature's wonders in a wilderness leads to respect and satisfaction with the environment (Chapter 6). Constructive use of discretionary time augments the QOL.

The Good Society

The structural features of a good society begin with an equalitarian framework. For motivation and production, a hierarchy is needed, but the QOL of the lower segments must be respected. Free markets for distribution of goods and services are recognized worldwide as essential for economic stability, as they most satisfactorily meet needs. Survival begins with maintaining health services of prevention and repair, avoiding man-made disasters, and protection from natural disasters. A social psychology of autonomy for ideas and beliefs, problem-solving intellectual activity, and freedom to find happiness will lead to the good society. Freedom, also, to express awe and wonder, spirituality and transcendence, free of dogma and authority is required. Respect for flora and fauna, for animals in their natural habitats, and the limits of Man's invasion of Nature are necessary if mankind is to adjust. Change in social structure and change in cultural patterns must be expected and guided into channels that benefit the majority. The ideal society will be built upon an educated populace, concerned with community issues and problems, that participates actively in its control. The four pillars envisioned by the European social quality study stand for the good society: social cohesion, inclusion, empowerment, and socioeconomic security. Internationally, institutions for security and peace should receive active support of nations.

Chapter 12
Interventions

> Know then thyself, presume not God to scan;
> The proper study of mankind is man.
> Plac'd on this isthmus of a middle state,
> A being darkly wise and rudely great:
> With too much knowledge for the sceptic side,
> With too much weakness for the stoic's pride,
> He hangs between, in doubt to act or rest;
> In doubt to deem himself a God or Beast
> Born but to die, and reas'ning but to err;
> Alike in ignorance, his reason such,
> Whether he thinks too little or too much;
> Chaos of thought and passion, all confus'd;
> Still by himself abus'd or disabus'd:
> Created half to rise and half to fall;
> Sole judge of truth, in endless error hurl'd;
> The glory, jest, and riddle of the world.
> *– Alexander Pope, Essay on Man, Epistle II.*

They (the Americans) have all a lively faith in the perfectibility of man, they judge that the diffusion of knowledge must necessarily be advantageous, and the consequences of ignorance fatal; they all consider society as a body in a state of improvement, humanity as a changing scene, in which nothing is, or ought to be, permanent; and they admit that what appears to them today to be good, may be superseded by something better tomorrow.
–Alexis de Tocqueville, Democracy in America (1835), Chap. 18.

Excellence depends on proper nutrition and health, self-discipline and self-restraint, the capacity to love and be loved; some measure of rationality, some aesthetic appreciation and some fulfillment of one's talents. Included in a good life is the development of moral relationships with others
–Paul Kurtz, "The Ethics of Secularism," FREE INQUIRY 28/5, Aug.-Sept., 2008.

In this review of interventions, let us examine some proposed interventions made by others and some of the means being employed to generate improvements in communities.

A.L. Ferriss, *Approaches to Improving the Quality of Life*, Social Indicators Research   117
Series 42, DOI 10.1007/978-90-481-9148-2_12, © Springer Science+Business Media B.V. 2010

Mukherjee

Ramkrishna Mukherjee summarized the thoughts of scholars who set forth valu-
ations on the QOL. The scholars were D. Meadows et al., *The Limits to Growth*,
M. Mesarovic and E. Pestel, *Mankind at the Turning Point*, A. Herrera et al.,
Catastrophe or a New Society?, and W. Leontief et al., *The Future of the World
Economy*. His summary included the following (Mukherjee, 1989, p. 85):

1. Zero population growth.
2. Zero industrial growth.
3. Absolute cost constraint of pollution control.
4. Nuclear power for energy generation.
5. Exploitation of costly resource materials.
6. Appropriate technological development for less-developed and developed
   countries, respectively.
7. Rapid agricultural growth in less-developed countries.
8. Maximum use of fossil fuels and solar power for energy generation.
9. Removal of income gap between less-developed and developed countries.
10. Removal of regional disparity in resource mobilization.

The generation of energy, per items four and eight above, is influenced by technological developments. Among them, wind power, wave power, and the tapping of
heat from below the earth's surface are being advocated as feasible solutions. Zero
population and industrial growth will require an ideology of slow growth and stability, leading to a world equilibrium. Number nine, the removal of the inequality of
income among nations, would entail policies that would transfer wealthier nations'
power to create wealth to less-developed nations. Stephen L. Parente (2008) has
pointed out that the barriers that constrain the transfer of technology need to be
removed in order to improve international competition. Implied in number nine is
a reduction in poverty, through reducing income disparities internationally. These
may be idealistic objectives to improve the QOL in the century ahead, but as population growth approaches 8 or 9 billion by mid-century, the need for such policies
will become more acceptable.

Community Forums on Social Indicators

Dulhy and Swartz (2006) have identified over 200 community indicators projects in
the United States. They have found factors making for organizational and political
success, and sometimes failure, of community forums. For success, they recommend establishing a conceptual framework for community indicators. They advise
that a theory be found that may explain variation in an indictor over time. A good
research design, they say, is needed if the results are to be respected by policymakers. They advise linking indicators to budgets and fiscal planning where possible.

In a discussion of political factors, the authors suggest promoting civic engagement of indicators. Indicator trends should be inclusive of government or private control. In seeking change in trend of an indicator, a community consensus is needed, rather than government or private control. "Raise money privately for the staff of an independent, tax exempt and non-partisan convener." Employ the media early in the process. They advise identifying a civic leader who will champion their efforts. It is important, they say, to achieve a success early, any success. Many other helpful suggestions are to be found in their article.

A program of community forums discussing current community issues has been organized in King County, Washington. Volunteers register as citizen counselors and agree to meet in groups of 4–12 persons to express opinions on community problems. One issue discussed, for example, was "Transportation: Public Priorities, Options and Funding." The groups' opinions are summarized and provided to the auditor's office. The purpose of the program is to encourage citizen participation, civic engagement, and citizenship education in government. Further information can be found at www.CountywideCommunityForums.org.

Other Interventions

Other initiatives include the following:

Building Educated Leaders for Life (BELL) was organized by Earl Martin Phalen in the 1990s to help underprivileged children attend college. Since then, many rising students have benefited from this program by attending college (Bornstein, 2007).

Gerald Chertavian in 1999 acquired a fortune by sale of a technology company. He established Year Up as an organization to help young underprivileged adults find careers in technology and science. Since beginning it, some 800 have graduated and entered higher education as basis for a career with investment and brokerage firms (Bornstein, 2007).

Another tactic involves engaging volunteers who devise steps to change particular conditions. The Jacksonville Community Council, Inc. (JCCI) assembles and publishes indicators, distributing to community organizations and leaders. They concern nine quality of life issues as follows: achieving educational excellence, sustaining a healthy community, growing a vibrant economy, maintaining responsive government, preserving the natural environment, moving around efficiently, promoting social well-being and harmony, keeping the community safe, enjoying arts, culture, and recreation. On these topics, social indicators are published and distributed in an annual Quality of Life Progress Report.

Study of trends in indicators has revealed interrelations among indicators. For example, an improvement in student achievement test scores has an influence on net employment growth. An increase in housing starts can negatively affect air quality by increasing traffic. Study of trends in indictors leads the JCCI to create Citizen Study Committees that focus upon a QOL topic, such as school dropouts or teen pregnancies. These volunteer study committees identify steps to modify the rate of change or direction of the prime indicator of the phenomena of interest. Their recommendations are evaluated by a policy study committee. Public awareness of the proposed steps is made by a citizen implementation task force. This may take several years. Eventually, the study process leads to action by citizen groups or agencies. Roles citizens play are characterized as stakeholders, advocates, framers, evaluators, and collaborators. The study, action, evaluation, etc. process takes time and the talents of many community citizens and agencies. The details of such a process and examples from cities are given in Epstein, Coates, Wray, and Swain (2006).

The community indicators program is summarized in *Results that Matter: Improving Communities by Engaging Citizens, Measuring Performance and Getting Things Done* by Paul D. Epstein, Paul M. Coates, Lyle D. Wray, and David Swain, published by John Wiley & Sons of 989 Market Street, San Francisco, CA, 94103-1741, in their Jossey-Bass imprint.

Southern Poverty Law Center

This organisation seeks to eliminate hate groups which employ violence to encroach upon the civil rights of others. Such encroachment depletes the QOL. One such organization is the Southern Poverty Law Center. Some of their activities are notable.

The Southern Poverty Law Center (The Center) of Montgomery, Alabama, is a nonprofit organization that publishes *Intelligence Report, SPLC Report, Teaching Tolerance* and other communications that give details of their activities. The approach is through legal action against groups that infringe upon the civil rights of others, as the accounts below will make clear.

In 2007, the Center initiated a lawsuit against Ron Edwards, leader of the Imperial Klans of America, for the beating in 2006 of Jordan Gruver, a 16-year old, at a county fair. The evidence of several witnesses was recorded in 2008. The SPLC won the case. Compensatory and punitive damages amounting to 2.5 million dollars were awarded to Gruver. Ron Edwards, the leader, is responsible for 1.5 million of the judgment. One of the jurors said, "It is the scariest thing to look at someone and know what evil is. When I looked at Mr. Edwards, that's what I saw."

Lists of hate groups are exposed by the Center. Recently, the racist activities of the Federation for Immigration Reform (FAIR) were documented. Receiving support from the Pioneer Fund, a hate group based in New York, FAIR agitates against undocumented immigrants, presumably because of their Latino and Catholic character. FAIR has operated since 1979, chiefly exhorting against "Latin onslaught" and is raising the fear of a possible race war between whites and Latinos. FAIR operates through field representatives, some with hate-group affiliations.

SPLC represented children with disabilities at schools in Louisiana, Mississippi, and Alabama. Out of this experience, it has organized a project in New Orleans,

School-to-Prison Reform Project, headed by Ron Lospennato. To insure that school children get the services and protection they need, SPLC initiates legal action, community activism, and lobbying. It estimates that nearly 100,000 children and teens are in custody, black youths being four times the number of white youths. Youth in the juvenile justice population suffer from learning disabilities and need educational services not normally provided them.

SPLC publishes material against hate crime. "Six Lessons from Jena" was distributed to 50,000 educators to inform them how to prevent racial tensions from generating violence in schools. The incident at the Jena High School in Louisiana concerned a 2006 beating of a white youth by six classmates. Originally charged as adults, the charges were reduced to second-degree battery and conspiracy charges. The court threw out the conviction of one lad because he should have been tried in juvenile court. The SPLC decried the incident but maintained that charges were excessive.

SPLC publishes the quarterly *Intelligence Report*, a magazine style report on hate and other groups that spread prejudice. The Spring 2008 issue featured "The Year of Hate," identifying many individuals and groups that advocate hatred against illegal immigrants, Hispanics, and others. It reported that hate groups increased to 926 in 2008, up from 888 in 2007, up from 844 in 2006. News items concerned neo-Nazis, racist skinheads, Ku Klux Klan, black separatists, white nationalists, Christian identity, neo-Confederate, and general hate groups. A map shows the state-by-state location of the groups. The issue contains articles describing activities of personalities that advocate hate against others. It lists hate groups and their website addresses. Each of these organizations threatens the well-being of others and thus challenges the security and living conditions of their QOL. In the interest of improving the QOL, hate groups should be nullified.

SPLC's work for justice, tolerance, and acceptance is supported by contributions. Since 1974, it has been developing an endowment which, in 2006, amounted to $192 million. It encourages supporters to join Partners for the Future, by including SPLC in wills.

SPLC is most effective in its legal action against hate groups.

Anti-defamation League

Another program striving to reduce prejudice is the Anti-Defamation League of New York City. It focuses on students in schools and colleges, providing anti-discrimination literature. It maintains a law enforcement program, instructing police officers in anti-bias training, extremism training, and the identification of hate crimes. Access to Law Enforcement Agency Resource Network is designed to help officers identify extremist activities. Its international program attempts to monitor anti-Semitism around the world and expose incidents and perpetrators. On the internet, it has a Hate Filter that blocks access to sites that advocate bigotry and violence toward groups on the basis of religious, racial, sexual orientation, or other personal characteristics. The program attempts to combat anti-Semitism and other forms of hatred. More information can be obtained on their website (www.adl.org).

Anti-materialism

The psychologist Tim Kasser presents arguments in his book, *The High Price of Materialism*, that "intrinsic values" should be substituted for our present materialism. Interestingly, Kasser identifies intrinsic values as consonant with the QOL domains in this book. With the QOL domains in parenthesis, this include "safe, secure" (Conservative), "competent" (Intellectual Autonomy), "worthy" (Mastery), "connected to others" (Social Acceptance), and "authentic and free" (Affective Autonomy). Kasser argues for personal change, family change, and societal change in order that intrinsic values be established. The material change is a change in values. In his book, he outlines specific steps to take in order to bring about change.

Economic Policies

Looking to changes in public policies to stimulate change and increase happiness, Layard (2005), also, emphasizes that values need to be changed. He would have us monitor the status of happiness in the population, and reassess our attitudes on numerous public issues. Being an economist, he is concerned over the world-wide poverty issue and would have prosperous nations contribute more to reducing poverty in less happy countries. In the health area, Layard singles out mental health as one of the most pressing current problems. As to family life, he would rearrange and improve the job–home relationship, including a provision for child care. He favors improving community life, reducing high unemployment, and prohibiting commercial advertising to children. All these changes are designed to enhance overall happiness. As an overriding key to improving society, Layard supports better education, both scientific and moral. Throughout his study, Layard advances the idea that happiness should be the criteria by which we should judge our policies and programs.

Religious bodies advance ideas to guide toward happiness and satisfaction with life, usually with a spiritual emphasis. The following are some of them.

Buddhism

Buddhists believe in a cycle of birth, life, death, and rebirth that continues until the soul is sufficiently perfect to enter nirvana. Life is suffering. To overcome it, one must follow the Four Noble Truths: the Truth of Suffering, the Truth of Arising, the Truth of Cessation, and the Truth of the Path.

In acknowledging that life is suffering, one is acknowledging life as it really is. Such is the first step toward happiness.

The Truth of Arising means that events are the consequence of a preceding cause. Desire causes rebirth in the world of suffering.

The Truth of Cessation represents the end of suffering when we overcome desires.

Finally, the Truth of the Path provides guidance for daily living. It consists of an Eightfold Path to follow in order to live a life that goes from suffering to rebirth and eventually to nirvana.

The Eightfold Path leads from suffering to happiness. The steps, not in any sequence, are the following: understanding, resolve, speech, action, livelihood, effort, mindfulness, and meditation. The path is not to be followed in any order, but it outlines the basic tasks of life. By following them, one divests ones' self of desire and suffering and eventually acquires happiness (Schoch, 2006).

Hinduism

Hindu theology consists of involved stories of actions of various gods, each representing a human tendency. The stories relate to enlightenment and happiness.

By following the discipline of yoga, one finds one's true identity. Yoga controls postures, movement, and breath, through which impulses are regulated and conquered. Different styles of yoga may be followed: the way of knowledge, the way of duty, and the way of life. These are the secrets of finding happiness: knowledge, duty, and love. These precepts are set forth in the *Bhagavad Gita*, a poem that originated about 300 BC. Our minds become clouded by delusions which must be discarded in order to be happy. Knowledge will make you happy, knowledge of your true self. One must act without concern for the outcome; one must be detached from the fruits of one's labor. Ganesha, the elephant, is a much beloved Hindu icon. Devotion to Ganesha brings happiness. A secret of happiness is found in detachment from "the world and its incessant demands (jinana yoga), action and its consequences (karma yoga), and the self and its ego-driven obsessions (bhakti yoga)." In freedom from desire lies happiness (Schoch, 2006).

Confucianism

Confucianism, a socio-political doctrine, is a complex system of social, political, philosophical, and religious thought. It strongly influences behavior in the Asian countries of China, Japan, Korea, Taiwan, Vietnam, and Singapore. Its teachings stress moral development in interpersonal relationships. The Chinese word *ren* may be variously translated as humanness, benevolence, supreme virtue, or the good. In the Burton Watson 2007 translation (New York: Columbia University Press) edition of *The Analytics,humanness* is the usual translation. From this is imputed a Confucian conception of the QOL: behavior is characterized by ethical values of trustworthiness, courtesy, respect, reciprocity, and loyalty. These are exercised through ritual, relationships with others, filial piety, and loyalty. Much is made of the proper behavior of "the gentleman." A gentleman is a perfect man, the ideal. A gentleman is morally correct, exhibits filial piety, is loyal to superiors, and cultivates humility and benevolence toward others. In his deportment, he is cordial, respectful, modest, deferential, and forthright (Book 1, #10). In Book 5, no. 16, the gentleman is characterized as prudent, respectful of superiors, and gives care for common people. In this, the gentleman follows the virtues set forth in the Equalitarian Commitment of the QOL. Happiness is not necessarily the result of good living conditions (Bk. 6, #11). Gods should be respected but kept at a distance (Bk. 6, #22).

In *The Analytics,* frequent mention is made of the importance of following "the Way," but nowhere is the Way defined, except as the virtuous life. One is told to follow the Way, practice humanness, and relax with the arts, which include music (Bk. 7, #6). The Golden Rule is negatively highlighted: "What you do not want others to do to you, do not do to others" (Bk 12, #2). Five qualities of humanness are emphasized (Bk. 17, #6): courtesy, tolerance, trustworthiness, diligence, and kindness. "Love of study" is also emphasized. Thus, the Confucian definition of the QOL is in terms of qualities of the virtuous man.

The Asian Barometer Surveys (ABS) conducted by Chuo University and the University of Tokyo provide the data to examine Confucianism in six east Asian societies: China, Japan, South Korea, Hong Kong, Singapore, and Taiwan (Inoguchi & Shin, 2009). In contrast to the Western world, Confucianism emphasizes family and community, discipline and hierarchy, consensus and harmony. This is in contrast to individualism, freedom and equality, and diversity and conflict – prominent values of the West. The surveys found that large majorities in the Confucian countries uphold the virtues of independence, diligence, honesty, mindfulness, and sincerity, while rejecting two non-Confucian virtues of religiosity and competitiveness. In fact, the virtues of first choice in the education of a child should be the following: in Japan, mindfulness (66%); in China, independence (48%); in Singapore, honesty (55%); in Hong Kong, honesty (41%); in Taiwan, diligence (45%); and in South Korea, sincerity (41%).

In China, where 56% of the population live in rural areas, the sense of well-being is high (Shu & Zhu, 2009). In western rural areas, the Chinese eat largely plant-based food. In consequence, heart disease and cancer are largely unknown, which is not the case along the eastern seaboard (Campbell & Campbell, 2004). Overall, the Chinese maintain a high level of satisfaction with interpersonal and marital relationships. Because of the prosperous economy, Chinese assess their present more favorably than their past. High economic growth promotes an optimistic outlook. Interpersonal relations are highly valued in China, coupled with a high marriage rate, leading to satisfaction with life. In their emphasis upon interpersonal relationships and marriage, the Chinese are following the advice of Confucius.

The most powerful influence upon the QOL in Japan is the marital status. Health stands high as a life concern, while the Japanese look negatively upon the social welfare system. The country has a large economy but currently experiences an economic downturn. This has affected the Japanese to be most satisfied with a post-material sphere of life and least satisfied with the public sphere. Lifestyle characteristics rated high by the Japanese include health, adequate food, spending time with the family, and being on good terms with others. These sources of satisfaction reflect the Confucian ideals (Inoguchi & Fuji, 2009).

South Korea for the last quarter century is being transformed into a modern state, though it continues to value many of the Confucian ideals: friendships, marriage, neighbors, family life, and health (Park, 2009). South Koreans are turning to materialistic values and are becoming less satisfied with them. Still, their QOL arises from marriage and their high standard of living. Some 56% rate themselves as happy. They find satisfaction in interpersonal relations and are least satisfied with the public sphere of their lives.

Christianity

According to the legacy of Thomas Aquinas (1224–1274), true happiness comes from contemplation of God. While some happiness is possible on earth, true happiness awaits in the afterlife. Wealth cannot make a person happy. The predominant effort of life should be the search for union with God, where supreme happiness may be found. Happiness cannot be found on earth, only in heaven. Christian virtues – justice, courage, temperance, and prudence, supported by faith, hope, and charity – are the foundation of earthly happiness that will lead to celestial happiness. The final step in attaining such happiness is God's grace.

As an example of the outreach of Christian bodies, Southern Baptist Convention, the largest Protestant denomination in America, reports numerous support activities other than missions to establish the church. A program of Human Needs Missions in Foreign Countries in 1995 supported more than 225 projects in 62 countries, costing 6 million dollars. The International Mission Board in 2006 supported World Hunger and Relief Ministries with 325 projects in 62 countries, costing $15 million. From a General Relief Fund, the Board provided help to areas devastated by tsunamis and storms in Southern Asia and the Indian Ocean, and in Alabama, Mississippi, and Louisiana. The Funds were applied to relieve hunger in Yugoslavia and drought-ridden African countries. Fifty-three children's homes in 183 community clinics were assisted. Some 46% of the general relief funds went to those suffering from natural disasters. This included hurricane victims in the Caribbean, victims of war in Chechnya, and flood victims in other areas of the world. Projects to enable people to help themselves involved "water, rural and urban development, vocational training and rehabilitation." In general, the program seeks to impact world hunger, disasters, relief, and development.

In addition, in 1995, a Program of Health Care Ministries in Foreign Centers supported more than 183,000 inpatients and more than two million outpatients. Programs were active in Paraguay, Indonesia, Ghana, Brazil, Venezuela, Korea, India, the Philippines, Gaza, Bolivia, Paraguay, the Dominican Republic, and other countries.

The motives for such extensive help to foreign peoples arise from the Christian missions of helping the less fortunate and converting people to their beliefs. The aim is to establish churches, ministers and church workers, and members. But along with churches, they build hospitals, community development programs, and poverty-reducing activities which benefit the QOL of natives (Rule, 2007).

Public Policies

In a wide-ranging essay on education and well-being, Michalos shows that education, represented as lifelong learning, impacts enormously on happiness. Public policies, then, to insure the well-being of its constituencies should invest in education of its citizens (Michalos, 2008).

The socialist system in Beijing, China, was the site for a survey of 732 persons examining perceived government accountability as influencing life satisfaction. The general hypothesis was supported: a person's perception of government accountability positively affects life satisfaction. An accountable government protects those with little social power. Citizens live in a politically powerless environment. However, the powerless attain satisfaction from government-supported economic and cultural features. Social power does not come from income; it derives from political influence. Religious people are politically powerless and marginal. The security of government accountability contributes to life satisfaction. These ideas reflect the socialist system in Beijing (Cheung & Leung, 2007).

In a study of 28 countries, the democratic system was found to provide the best environment for happiness, after controlling for sociodemocratic and other cultural factors. The relationship to happiness was stronger in more mature than recent democratic systems. The study concluded that higher levels of democracy lead to policies and procedures that reflect people's preferences and thus to satisfaction and happiness (Dorn, Fischer, Kirchgassner, & Sousa-Poza, 2007).

The Mayo Clinic

A major medical facility in Rochester, Minnesota, the Mayo Clinic has produced and distributed a pamphlet *Live Longer, Live Better*. It discusses seven topics for the betterment of the QOL: (1) stay physically active; (2) exercise your mind; (3) make your health a priority; (4) do not smoke; (5) invest in the major relationships of your life; (6) take time for the things you enjoy; (7) stay connected to your community. The discussion includes accounts of the activities of the Clinic's physicians and staff.

These rules for good health are offered in other medical newsletters, for example, those issued by the Harvard University Medical School and Duke University Medical School.

The Government in Industrial Democracies

Is the welfare state more conducive to life satisfaction and happiness than other forms of industrial democracy? Pacek and Radcliff (2008) examined life satisfaction and happiness in 18 modern industrial democracies, including a measure reflecting the welfare state dimension. Using the World Values Survey, 1981–2000, they concluded that the welfare state has a positive and significant impact upon happiness and life satisfaction. It appears that the insecurity of market forces acts negatively on satisfaction and happiness; but imposing security by the welfare state restores it.

R. Estes (2007) constructed an Index of Social Progress. Ten factors are known to be valid indicators of social development: education, health status, women's status, defense effort, economic, demographic, environmental, social chaos, cultural diversity, and welfare effort. Several indicators are included for each of these domains, 40 altogether. He assembled data for 31 countries considered to be in transition. What has stimulated social progress over recent decades? Between 1970 and 1990, the drawbacks were political corruption, infectious and communicable diseases, plus depredation of the landscape. Between 1990 and 2000, Latin American countries experienced net social losses of about 4%. States of Central and Eastern Europe, 1990–2000, showed high average progress scores. They had high levels of social protection, were reverting to private ownership, and a change in socio-political ideologies contributed to their progress. The Baltic States, likewise, progressed with their transition to a market economy and more "transparent" political systems. Countries of the Russian Federation are at a comparatively high level of social development. Dynamic private economies are emerging. But, these countries are experiencing social chaos that retards progress, and they score lower than the Baltic States on environmental pollution and the status of women. Their level of expenditure on defense continues high. Estes' report also evaluates other areas and countries, but the results of his analysis of the progress of nations supports the notion that transforming the nations to more open, competitive, transparent, and "people centered" socioeconomic systems leads to progress. Privatization of enterprises contributes to progress, as opposed to inefficient state enterprises. Some of the countries had benefited from eleemosynary contributions of the Gates, Turner, and Soros foundations (Ross, 2007).

Foundations

In most of the world, needs are satisfied for the QOL through the free market system. It operates upon norms and values that uphold private property, respect for contracts, and honesty in dealings. In the process, profit accrues. The government taxes excess profits but allows profits to be free of taxes if the money is used for charitable purposes or other benefits to society. Consequently, money is contributed to foundations where it is used for programs that improve the human condition or otherwise benefits society. Now, almost all communities have foundations that contribute to the QOL of the community. Many, however, are national and international in scope. The 25 largest are herewith listed with their capital accumulations:

Bill and Melinda Gates Foundation, USA, $35.9 billion.
Wellcome Trust, England, $26.4 billion.
Howard Hughes Medical Institute, USA, $18.6 billion.
Ford Foundation, USA, $13.7 billion.
The Church Commissioners of England, England, $10.5 billion.
J. Paul Getty Trust, USA, $10.1 billion.
Li Ka Shing Foundation, Hong Kong, $10.0 billion.
Robert Wood Johnson Foundation, USA, $10.0 billion.
William and Flora Hewlett Foundation, USA, $8.5 billion.
W. K. Kellogg Foundation, USA, $8.4 billion.
Lilly Endowment, USA, $7.6 billion.
Garfield Foundation, England, $6.9 billion.
Robert Bosch Foundation, Germany, $6.9 billion.
David and Lucile Packard Foundation, USA, $6.3 billion.
Andrew W. Mellon Foundation, USA, $6.1 billion.
John D. and Catherine T. McArthur Foundation, USA, $6.1 billion.
Realdania, Denmark, $5.6 billion.
Knut and Alice Wallenberg Foundation, Sweden, $5.3 billion.
The California Endowment, USA, $4.4 billion.
The Pew Charitable Trust, USA, $4.1 billion.
'Calouste Gulbenkian Foundation, Portugal, $3.8 billion.
Rockefeller Foundation, USA, $3.8 billion.
The Starr Foundation, USA, $3.5 billion.
The Kresge Foundation, USA, $3.3 billion.
The purposes of these and other foundations may be found on their websites or, for US foundations, in *The Foundation Directory* issued by the Russell Sage Foundation.

To illustrate the scope and impact of foundation donations, the major programs of the Bill and Melinda Gates Foundation, which was doubled in size when Warren Buffett donated to it, includes a global health program and programs in the area of global development, which include financial services for the poor, agricultural development, global libraries, and global special initiatives. Its US program includes libraries and educational services in the Pacific Northwest. It also has a program labeled Lifespan. The foundation contributes assistance when disasters occur, such as the Indian Ocean Earthquake and the Kashmir earthquake (Bell, 1999).

There is also a *Random Acts of Kindness Foundation*. Its mission is to inspire people to practice kindness and pass the idea on to others. Its website provides educational and community ideas, guidance, a newsletter, lesson plans for teachers, and other inspirational communications. It sends a delegate to the World Kindness Movement, an international organization that promotes kindness and compassion in various countries. More information may be found on www.actsofkindness.org.

The Foundation for a Better Life (www.forbetterlife.org) encourages adoption of values that reflect personal accountability. Its message is broadcast through various media, such as posters or billboards, television, outdoor advertising. Examples of the values the Foundation encourages are Appreciation, Compassion, Doing the Right Thing, Friendship, Helping Others, Integrity, Love, Loyalty, Responsibility, Self-esteem, Tolerance, and others. It does not accept donations. It believes that individuals who take responsibility for their behavior will take care of family, job, community, and country. Its website carries additional information.

Interventions

Interventions that have been identified, domain by domain, in this volume are here summarized.

Organization and Policy

Change in dietary habits from meat to vegetables and fruit will reduce environmental pollution and reduce global warming.

Energy will be conserved when buildings are made more energy efficient.

Legal action against hate groups effectively reduces this source of violence.

Religious groups should reduce interfaith friction and extend tolerance toward others.

The Security Council of the United Nations seeks to maintain peace.

Neighborhoods of homogeneous people foster social support and group participation.

Low interest loans from small village banks lead to independence and private gain.

Norms and values supporting income transfer from the upper to lower segments of income distribution will lead to reducing income inequality. Such a revision of the economic system will move toward better QOL, as in some European countries.

Communities may improve family life by offering a conflict resolution service.

Legal restrictions on carbon dioxide and other emissions are needed in order to reduce greenhouse gases and restore a normal climate.

Communities and corporations should establish sustainable energy sources from wind, waves, water, and other such forces.

The nation should take steps to reduce poverty and expand the middle class.

Police should be trained to identify hate crime incidents and perpetrators.

Stimulating creativity through education and arts will reduce crime and conflict.

Leaders should reinforce norms of morality and justice in the community.

A better QOL will evolve from a good society structured for equality and justice.

For the improvement and production of "love-energy," increase the creative heroes of love and of the heroes of Truth and Beauty; increase generation of love by rank and file of people and of groups and institutions, and of cultures.

Interpersonal

Conflict resolution process benefits contending parties by reducing hostility.

Most religious bodies advocate justice, mercy, equity, and consideration of others.

Steps to better mental health involve developing self-assurance through leisure time activities, resolving family problems, being socially inclusive, and developing a secure self-concept.

In socializing the child, build self-confidence in a harmonious family setting.

Negative emotions are part of life. Accommodate to them through discipline.

With a tranquil state of mind, seek happiness of others rather than seeking happiness for yourself.

Income beyond that needed for basic necessities will not expand happiness.

Attitude change results from applying proven psychological principles (Chapter 4).

The free exercise of capabilities results in creative, artistic, and intellectual attainments.

Eating nutritious food and exercising regularly leads to better health and QOL.

References

Abbey, A., & Andres, F. M. (1986). Modeling the psychological determinants of life quality. In M. A. Frank (Ed.), *Research on the quality of life*. Ann Arbor, MI: The University of Michigan Press.

Al-Anon. (1995). *How Al-Anon works for families and friends of alcoholics*. Virginia Beach, VA: Al-Anon Family Group Headquarters, Inc.

Albrecht, D. E., & Albrecht, C. M. (2007). Income inequality: The influence of economic structure and social conditions. *Sociological Spectrum, 27*(2), 165–182.

Alsker, K., Moen, B. E., & Kristoffersen, K. (2008, May). Health-related quality of life among abused women one year after leaving a violent partner. *Social Indicators Research, 86*(3).

Anderson, J. P., Kaplan, R. M., & Smith, C. W. (2004). Arthritis impact on U. S. life quality: Morbidity and mortality effects from national health Interview survey data 1986–1988 and 1994 using QWSBX1 estimates of well-being. *Social Indicators Research, 69*(1).

Augsberger, D. (1992). *Conflict mediation across cultures*. Louisville: Westminister/John Knox Press.

Baker, D. A., & Palmer, R. J. (2006). Examining the effects of perceptions of community and recreation participation on the quality of life. *Social Indicators Research, 75*(3).

Baker, S. (2009, April). Building a better brain. *Discover.*

Ball, R., & Cheova, K. (2008, September). Absolute income, relative income, and happiness. *Social Indicators Research, 88*(3).

Baumbaugh-Smith, J., Gross, H., Wollman, N., & Yoder, B. (2008, February). NIVAH: A composite index measuring violence and health in the U. S. *Social Indicators Research, 85*(3).

Baumeister, R. F., & Tenge, J. M. (2003). The social self. In T. Millon & M. J. Lerner (Eds.), *Personality and Social Psychology*. In T. B. Weiner (ed. in chief), *Handbook of psychology* (Vol. 5, pp. 332–334). Hoboken, NJ: John Wiley & Sons, Inc.

Barstad, A. (2008, May). Explaining changing suicide rates in Norway 1948–2004: The role of social integration. *Social Indicators Research, 87*(1).

Bell, W. (1999). *Humanity 3000 seminar No. 2 proceedings* (p. 15). Leavenworth, WA: Foundation for the Future.

Benson, H. (1996). *Timeless healing: The power and biology of belief.* New York: Scribners.

Berman, Y., & Philips, D. (2000). Indicators of social quality and social exclusion at national and community level. *Social Indicators Research 50*, 329–350.

Bhui, K., King, M., Dein, S., & O'Connor, W. (2008). Ethnicity and religious coping with mental distress. *Journal of Mental Health, 17*(2), 141–151.

Bjornskov, C. (2008, March). Social capital and happiness in the United States. *Applied Research in Quality of Life, 3*(1).

Bockerman, P., & Ilmakunnas, P. (2006). Elusive effects of unemployment on happiness. *Social Indicators Research, 79*(1).

Bohnke, P. (2008, June). Does society matter? Life satisfaction in the enlarged Europe. *Social Indicators Research, 87*(2).

Bonikowski, B., & McPherson, M. (2006) The sociology of voluntary associations. In C. D. Bryant & D. L. Peck (Eds.), *21st century sociology* (Vol. 1). Thousand Oaks, CA: Sage Publications

Bornstein, D. (2007, November/December). Pursuing happiness. *The World Ark,* pp 10–16.

Bramston, P., Pretty, G., & Chipuer, H. (2002). Unraveling subjective quality of life: An investigation of individual and community determinants. *Social Indicators Research, 59*(3).

Bronisch, T. (2001). Suicide. In N. J. Smelser & P. B. Bates (Eds.), *International encyclopedia of the social and behavioral sciences* (Vol. 22). New York: Elsevier.

Broome, J. (2008). The ethics of climate change. *Scientific American, 298*(6).

Brulde, B. (2007). Happiness and the good life: Special issue. *Journal of Happiness Studies,* 8(1).

Burgio, A., Murrianni, L., & Folino-Gallo, P. (2009). Differences in life expectancy and disability free life expectancy in Italy: A challenge to health systems. *Social Indicators Research, 92*(1).

Buscaglia, L. (1972). *Love.* New York: Ballantine Books, division of Random House.

Campbell, T. C., & Campbell II, T. M. (2004). *The China study.* Dallas, TX: Beneella Books.

Carle, A. C., Bauman, K. J., & Short, K. (2009). Assessing the measurement and structure of material hardship in the United States. *Social Indicators Research, 92*(1).

Cassidy, J. (2000, February 7). The price prophet. *The New Yorker,* pp. 44–51.

Chan, J., Ho-Pong, T., & Chan, E. (2006). Reconsidering social cohesion: Developing a definition and analytical framework for empirical research. *Social Indicators Research,* 75(2).

Chen, C. (2003). Revisiting the disengagement theory with differentials in the determinants of life satisfaction. *Social Indicators Research, 64*(2).

Cheung, C.-K., & Leung, K.-K. (2007, July). Enhancing life satisfaction by government accountability in China. *Social Indicators Research, 82*(3).

Cheung, C.-K., & Leung, K.-K. (2008). Retrospective and prospective evaluations of environmental quality under urban renewal as determinants of residents' subjective quality of live. *Social Indicators Research,* 85(2).

Cicognani, E., Pirini, C., Keyes, C., Joshanloo, M., Rostami, R., & Nosratabadi, M. (2008, October). Social participation, sense of community and social well-being: A study of American, Italian and Iranian University students. *Social Indicators Research, 89*(1).

Cornelisse-Vermaat, Judith, R., Antonides, Van Ophem, G. J. A. C., & Van Den Brink, H. M. (2006, October). Body mass index, perceived health, and happiness: Their determinants and structural relationships. *Social Indicators Research, 79*(1).

Coser, L. A. (1956). *The Functions of social conflict.* Glencoe: The Free Press.

Coser, L. A. (1961). The termination of conflict. *Journal of Conflict Resolution, 5,* 347–353

Cottrell, G., Weldon, M., & Mulligan, S. (2008, May). Measuring changes in family wellbeing in New Zealand 1981–2001. *Social Indicators Research, 86*(3).

Cramer, V., Torgersen, S., & Krignglen, E. (2004). Quality of life in a city: The effect of population density. *Social Indicators Research, 69*(1).

Cummins, R. A. (1996). The domains of life satisfaction: An attempt to order chaos. *Social Indicators Research,* 38(3), 303–328.

Cummins, R. A. (2000). Objective and subjective quality of life, an interactive model. *Social Indicators Research, 52*(1).

Cummins, R. A., Eckersley, R., Pallant, J., van Vugt, J., & Misajon, R. (2003). Developing a national index of subjective well-being: The Australian unity well-being index. *Social Indicators Research, 64*(2).

Dalai L., His Holiness the 14th, & Howard C. C. (1999). *The art of happiness: A handbook for living.* London: Hodder and Soughton, Ltd.

Dees, M. (2007, May 28). *Hate groups and hate activity* (letter). Montgomery, AL: Southern Poverty Law Center.

Delamonnica, E. E., & Minujin, A. (2007). Incidence, depth and severity of children in poverty. *Social Indicators Research, 82*(2).

de Waal, Frans, B. M. (2006) Primates and Philosophers, Princeton: University Press.

Diamond, J. (2005). *Collapse.* New York: Penguin Group.

Diener, E. (1995). A value based index for measuring national quality of life. *Social Indicators Research, 36,* 107–127.

Diener, E. (2005). Guidelines for national indicators of subjective well-being and ill-being. *SINET,* *84*(Nov), 4–6.

Diener, E., & Suh, E. (1997). Measuring the quality of life: Economic, social and subjective indicators. *Social Indicators Research, 40*, 189–216.

Dorn, D., Fischer, J. A., Kirchgassner, G., & Sousa-Poza, A. (2007, July). Is it culture democracy? The impact of democracy and culture on happiness. *Social Indicators Research, 82*(3).

Dulhy, M., & Swartz, N. (2006, October). Connecting knowledge and policy: The promise of community indicators. *Social Indicators Research, 79*(1).

Durkheim, E. (2002). *Suicide.* London and NY: P Rudledge.

Dyette, J. (2006). Winds of change. *Catalyst, 5*(2), 2–3.

Eagly, A. H. (2000). Attitude change. In A. E. Kazdin (Ed.), *Encyclopedia of psychology* (Vol. 1). New York: Oxford University Press.

Easterlin, R. A. (1974). Does economic growth improve the human lot. In P. A. David & M. W. Reeder (Eds.), *Nations and households in economic growth: Essays in honor of moses Abramowitz.* New York: Academic Press.

Eid, M., & Diener, E. (2004). Global judgments of subjective well-being: Situational variability and long-term stability. *Social Indicators Research, 65*(3).

Ellison, C. G., & Fan, D. (2008, September). Daily spiritual experiences and psychological well-being among U. S. adults. *Social Indicators Research, 88*(2).

Epstein, P. D., Coates, P. M., Wray, L. D., & Swain, D. (2006). *Results that matter: Improving communities by engaging citizens, measuring performance, and getting things done.* San Francisco: Jossey-Bass.

Esselstyn, C. B., Jr., (2007). *Prevent and reverse heart disease.* New York: Penguin Group.

Estes, R. (2007, September). Development challenges and opportunities confronting economies in transition. *Social Indicators Research, 83*(3).

Fandrem, H., San, D. K., Roland, E. (2009). Depressive symptoms among native and immigrant adolescents in Norway: The role of gender and urbanization. *Social Indicators Research, 92*(1).

Federal Trade Commission (2009). *Taking charge: Fighting back against identity theft, pamphlet.* Washington, DC: Federal Trade Commission.

Felsitner, W. L., Abel, R. L., & Sarat, A. (1980–1981). The emergence and transformation of disputes: Naming, blaming, claiming. *Law and Society Review*, 15(3–4): 631–654.

Ferrara, A. (2001), Person and Self: Philosophical aspects, In J. S. Neil & B. B. Paul (Eds.), *International encyclopedia of the social and behavioral sciences* (Vol. 16). New York: Elsevier

Ferriss, A. L. (1990). The quality of life in the United States. *SINET 21,* 1–6.

Ferriss, A. L. (1999). A note on happiness, money and time. *SINET 57,* 8.

Ferriss, A. L. (2000). The quality of life among U. S. states. *Social Indicators Research, 49,* 1–23.

Ferriss, A. L. (2001). The domains of the quality of life. *Bulletin de Methodologie Sociologique, 72,* 5–1

Ferriss, A. L. (2006). Social structure and child poverty. *Social Indicators Research, 78*(2).

Forni, P. M. (2002). *Choosing civility.* New York: St. Martin's Griffin.

Fuhrman, J. (1999). *Discover the health equation.* Fuhrman.

Fuhrman, J. (2003). *Eat to live.* Boston, London: Little, Brown and Co.

Fuhrman, J. (2004). *Cholesterol protection for life.* Flemington, New Jersey: Fuhrman.

Gomes, P. J. (2002). *The Good Life,* San Francisco: Harper San Francisco.

Gorgellis, Y., Tsitsianis, N., & Yin, Y. (2009). Personal values as mitigating factors in the link between income and life satisfaction: Evidence from the European social survey. *Social Indicators Research, 91*(3).

Green, J. J., Kerstetter, K., & Nylander III, A. B. (2008). Socioeconomic resources and self-rated health: A study in the Mississippi Delta. *Sociological Spectrum, 28*(2).

Green, R. G. (1999). *Human aggression* (2nd ed.). Buckingham, Philadelphia: Open University Press.

Gilbert, D. (2006). *Stumbling on happiness.* New York: Alfred A. Knopf.

Gill, D. A. (2007, November–December). Secondary trauma or secondary disaster? Insights from hurricane Katrina. *Sociological Spectrum, 27*(6).

Giuffre, P., Dellinger, K. & Williams, C. L. (2008). No retribution for being gay: Inequality in gay-friendly workplaces. *Sociological Sectrum, 28*(3).

Glatzer, W. (2001). German sociologists are looking for the 'good society'. *Social Indicators Research, 55,* 35–359.

Grant, J. T. (2008, September–October). Measuring aggregate religiosity in the United States, 1952–2005. *Sociological Spectrum, 28*(5).

Grigg, A. F. (1996). Fear. *Encyclopedia Americana, 11,* 61–62.

Gronlund, L. (2008, Spring). Nuclear power in a warming world. *Catalyst, 7*(1).

Groot, W., & ven den Brink, H. M. (2003, January). Sympathy and the value of health: The spillover effects of migraine and household well-being. *Social Indicators Research, 61*(1).

Hagerty, M. R., & Veenhoven, R. (2003), Wealth and happiness revisited: Growing national income does go with greater happiness. *Social Indicators Research, 64,* 1–27.

Hagerty, M. R., & Veenhoven, R. (2006). Rising happiness in nations 1946–2004: A reply to Easterlin. *Social Indicators Research, 79*(3), 421–436.

Hagerty, M. R., Cummins, R., Ferriss, A. L., Land, K., Michalos, A. C., Peterson, M., et al. (2000). Quality of life indices for national policy: Review and agenda for research. *Social Indicators Research, 76,* 343–366.

Hajiran, H. (2006). Toward a quality of life theory: Net domestic product of happiness. *Social Indicators Research, 75*(1).

Haller, M., & Hadler, M. (2006). How social relations and structures can produce happiness and unhappiness: An international comparative analysis. *Social Indicators Research, 75*(2).

Hansen, J. (2007, May 7). Why we can't wait: a 5-step plan for solving the global crisis. *The Nation.*

Harris, M. (2007, April). Measuring optimism in South Africa. *Social Indicators Research, 81*(2), April.

Harris, S. (2004). *The end of faith.* New York: W. W. Norton & Co.

Harvey, A. S., & Mukhopadhyay, A. K. (2007). When twenty-four hours is not enough: Time poverty of working parents. *Social Indicators Research, 82,* 57–77.

Haub, C. (2002). 2002 World population data sheet. Washington, DC: The Population Reference Bureau.

Headey, B. (2008a, April). Life goals matter to happiness: A revision of set-point theory. *Social Indicators Research, 86*(2).

Headey, B. (2008b, October). Poverty is low consumption and low wealth, not just low income. *Social Indicators Research, 89*(1).

Headey, B., Muffels, R., & Wooden, M. (2008, May). Money does not buy happiness: Or does it? A reassessment based on the combined effects of wealth, income and consumption. *Social Indicators Research, 87*(1).

Heinsohn, G. (2001). Genocide: Historical aspects. In J. S. Neil & P. B. Bates (Eds.), *International encyclopedia of the social and behavioral sciences* (Vol. 9). New York: Elsevier.

Helliwell, J. F. (2007). Wekk-being and social capital: Does suicide pose a puzzle. *Social Indicators Research, 81*(3).

Herrman, M. (Ed.) (1994). Introduction. In M. S. Herrman (Ed.), *Resolving conflict: Strategies for local government.* Washington, DC: International City/Country Management Association.

Herrman, M. (Ed.) (2005). *The blackwell handbook of mediation: Building theory, research and practice.* Oxford: Blackwell.

Hijab, N. (2007). Hunger: The world's biggest killer. *Cosmos Bulletin, 60* (7–8).

Hummer, R. A., Rogers, R. G., Nam, C. B., & Elison, C. G. (1999). Religious involvement and U. S. adult mortality. *Demography, 36*(2), 273–285.

Huppert, F. A., Marks, N., Clark, A., Siegrist, J., Stutzer, A., Vitterso, J., et al. (2009). Measuring the well-being across Europe: Description of the ESS well-being module and preliminary findings. *Social Indicators Research, 91*(3).

Huschka, D., & Mau, S. (2006). Social anomie and racial segregation in South Africa. *Social Indicators Research, 76*(3).

Hutchinson, E. D. (1949). *How to think creatively*. New York and Nashville, TN: Abingdon Press.

Ig, Y.-K. (2008). Environmentally responsible happy nation index: Towards an internationally acceptable national success indicator. *Social Indicators Research, 85*(3).

Inoguchi, T., & Fuji, S. (2009, June). The quality of life in Japan. *Social Indicators Research, 92*(2).

Inoguchi, T., & Shin, D. C. (2009, June). The quality of life in Confucian Asia: From physical welfare to subjective well-being. *Social Indicators Research, 92*(2).

Iwasaki, Y. (2007). Leisure and quality of life in an international and multicultural context: What Are major pathways linking leisure to quality of life? *Social Indicators Research, 81*(1).

Iwasaki, Y. (2007). Leisure and the quality of life in an international and multicultural context: What are major pathways linking leisure to quality of life? *Social Indicators Research, 82*(2).

Jai, H., Lubetkin, E. I., Moriarty, D. G., & Zack, M. M. (2007). A comparison of healthy days and EuroQol EQ-5D measures in two US adult samples. *Applied Research in Quality of Life, 2*(3).

Joseph, J. (2003). *Social theory*. Edinburgh: Edinburgh University Press.

Joshanloo, M., & Nosratabadi, N. (2009). Levels of mental health continuum and mental health traits. *Social Indicators Research, 90*(2).

Kafetsios, K. (2006). Social support and well-being in contemporary Greek society: Examination of multiple indicators of different levels of analysis. *Social Indicators Research, 76*(1).

Kahneman, D., Krueger, A. B., Schkade, D., Schwartz, N., & Stone, A. (2004, May). Toward national well-being accounts. *American Economic Association Papers and Proceedings, 94*(2), 429–434.

Kaplan, R. M., Anderson, J. P., & Kaplan, C. M. (2006, March). Modeling quality-adjusted life expectancy loss resulting from tobacco use in the United States. *Social Indicators Research, 81*(1).

Kaplan, S. (2008, August). The discover interview, Phil Brown. *Discover.*

Kashner, Z. (2007). *The world almanac and book of facts 2007*. New York: World Almanac Books.

Kauer, J., & Rubman, A. L. (2007). *Obesity can be deadly, more ultimate healing*. Stanford, CT: Bottom Line Books.

Keyes, C. L. M. (1998). Social well-being. *Social Psychology Quarterly, 61*(2), 121–140.

Keyes, C. L. M. (2006). Subjective well-being in mental health and human development research worldwide: An introduction. *Social Indicators Research, 77*(1).

Kim, Myoung So, Hye Won Kim, Kyoeong Ho Cha & Jeeyoung Lim, (2007). What makes Koreans happy? Exploration on the structure of happy life among Korean adults. *Social Indicators Research, 82*(2), 265–286.

Kraus, S., & Sears, S. (2009). Measuring the immmeasurables: Development and initial validation of the self-other four immeasurables (SOFI) scale based on Buddhist teaching on loving kindness, compassion, joy and equanimity. *Social Indicators Research,* 92(1).

Kyokai, Bukkyo Dendo (Buddhist Printing Foundation) (1990). *The teaching of Buddha*. Tokyo, Japan: Bukkyo Dendo Kyokai.

Lai, Johanna Hiu-Wai, Michael Harris Bond, & Natalie Hung-Hung Hui (2007). The role of social axioms in predicting life satisfaction: A longitudinal study in Hong Konng. *Social Indicators Research, 81*(1).

Land, K. C. (2005). Daniel Kahneman and colleagues on national well-being accounts. *SINET, 84*(Nov), 1–3.

Laurer, R. H. & Laurer, J. E. (2006). *Social problems and the quality of life* (10th ed.). New York: McGraw Hill.

Layard, R. (2005). *Happiness*. New York: The Penguin Press.

Lee, D. Y., Park, S. H. M., Uhlemann, R., & Patsula, P. (2000). What makes you happy? A comparison of self-reported criteria of happiness between two cultures. *Social Indicators Research, 50*(3), 351–362.

Liao, P.-S. (2009). Parallels between objective indicators and subjective perceptions of quality of life: A study of metropolitan and county areas in Taiwan. *Social Indicators Research, 91*(1).

Lin, C.-H., & Yang, C.-h. (2009). An analysis of educational inequality in Taiwan after the higher education expansion. *Social Indicators Research, 90*(2).

Marks, G. N. (2008). Are father's or mother's socioeconomic characteristics more important influences on student's performance? Recent international evidence. *Social Indicators Research, 85*(2).

Marsa, L. (2008, June). The acid test. *Discover.*

Matras, J. (1977). *Introduction to population.* Edgewood Cliffs, NJ: Prentice Hall, Inc.

Mazumdar, K. (2000). Causal flow between human well-being and per capita real gross domestic product. *Social Indicators Research, 50*(3).

McAuliffe, K. (2008, September). Mental fitness. *Discover.*

McAuliffe, K. (2009). Are we still evolving? *Discover,* March

McNicoll, G. (2001). Fertility: Institutional and political approaches. In N. J. Spenser & P. B. Bates (Eds.), *International encyclopedia of the social and behavioral sciences* (Vol. 8). New York: Elsevier.

Michalos, A. (2008, July). Education, happiness and wellbeing. *Social Indicators Research, 87*(3).

Michalos, A. (2003, January). Policing services and the quality of life. *Social Indicators Research, 61*(1).

Michalos, A., & Zumbo, B. D. (2000). Criminal victimization and the quality of life. *Social Indicators Research, 50*(3).

Michalos, A., & Zumbo, B. D. (2002). Healthy days, health satisfaction and satisfaction with the overall quality of life. *Social Indicators Research, 59*(3).

Mohr, S. (2009, April–May). Exposing the myth of alcoholics anonymous. *Free Inquiry, 29*(3).

Moller, V. (2007). Quality of life in South Africa – The first ten years of democracy. *Social Indicators Research, 81*(2), 181–201.

Monnickendam, M., & Berman, Y. (2008, May). An empirical analysis of the interrelationship between components of the social quality theoretical construct. *Social Indicators Research, 86*(3).

Moore, K. A., Vandivere, S., & Redd, Z. (2006). A sociodemographic risk index. *Social Indicators Research, 75*(1).

Moriarty, D. G. (2007). *Health and the quality of life: Population perspectives.* Paper presented at the April 11–14, 2007 annual meeting of the Southern Sociological Society, Atlanta, GA: Centers for Disease Control and Prevention.

Moss, M. (1999). *Welfare dimensions of productivity management, measurement and implementation of productivity.* Washington, DC: National Academy of Sciences.

Muhajarine, N., Labonte, R., Williams, A., & Randall, J. (2008, January). Person, perception, and place what matters to health and quality of life. *Social Indicators Research, 85*(1).

Mukherjee, R. (1989). *The quality of life: Valuation in social research.* New Delhi/Newbury Park/London: Sage Publications.

Naimark, N. M. (2001). History of ethnic clensing. In N. J. Smelser & P. B. Bates (Eds.), *International encyclopedia of social and behavioral sciences* (Vol. 7). New York: Elsevier.

Nam, C. B. (1994). *Understanding population change.* Itasca, IL: F. E. Peacock, Inc.

National Center for Health Statistics (2003). *Health, United States 2003.* Hyattesville, MD: National Center for Health Statistics.

National Center for Health Statistics (2005). *Health, United States 2005.* Hyattsville, MD: National Center for Health Statistics.

Neira, I., Vazquez, E., & Portela, M. (2009). An empirical analysis of social capital and economic growth in Europe (1980–2000). *Social Indicators Research, 92*(1).

Nieminen, T., Martelin, T., Koskinen, S., Simpura, J., Alanen, E., & Harkanen, T., et al. (2008, February). Measurement and socio-demographic variation of social capital in a large population-based survey. *Social Indicators Research, 85*(3).

Nkwocha, E. E. (2009). Water supply deficiency and implications for rural development in the Niger-Delta region of Nigeria. *Social Indicators Research, 90*(3).

Nordstrom, C. R. (2001). War: Anthropological aspects. In N. J. Smelser & P. B. Baltes (Eds.), *International encyclopedia of the social and behavioral sciences*. New York: Elsevier.

Nowak, A., Vollacher, R. R., & Miller, M. E. (2003). Social influence and group dynamics. In T. Millon & M. J. Lerner (Eds.), *Personality and social psychology* (Vol. 5). In T. B. Weiner (Ed. in chief), *Handbook of psychology*. Hoboken, NJ: John Wiley & Sons, Inc.

O'Neil, B., & Balk, D. (2001). World population futures. *Population Bulletin, 56*(3).

Pacek, A. C., & Radcliff, B. (2008, October). Welfare policy and subjective well-being across nations: An individual-level assessment. *Social Indicators Research, 89*(1).

Parente, S. L. (2008). Narrowing the economic gap in the 21st century. In R. H. Kim, E. J. Fulner, & M. A. O'Grady (Eds.), *2008 Index of economic freedom*. Washington, DC: The Heritage Foundation and Dow Jones & Co., Inc.

Park, C.-M. (2009, June). The quality of life in South Korea. *Social Indicators Research, 92*(2).

Parker, L. (2007, April 11). Klan-busters fighting on a new front. *USA Today*.

Pichler, F. (2006). Subjective quality of life of young Europeans: Felling happy but who knows why? *Social Indicators Research, 75*(3).

Pollard, E. L., & Lee, P. D. (2003, January). Child well-being: A systematic review of the literature. *Social Indicators Research, 61*(1).

Prentice, D. A. (2000). Values. In A. E. Kazdin (ed.), *Encyclopedia of psychology* (Vol. 8) New York: Oxford University Press.

Ratzabm S. C., Filerman, G. L., & Sar, J. W. (2000, March). Attaining global health: Challenges and opportunities. *Population Bulletin, 55*(1).

Ravanera, Z. (2007). Informal networks social capital of fathers: What does the social engagement survey tell us? *Social Indicators Research, 83*(2).

Requena, F. (2003, March). Social capital, satisfaction and quality of life in the workplace. *Social Indicators Research, 61*(3).

Ricard, M. (2000, March 7). *L'infini dans la paume de la main*. Paris: Nil Editions.

Richie, L. A., & Gill, D. A. (2007, January–February) Social capital theory as an integrating theoretical framework in technological disaster research. *Sociological Spectrum, 27*(1), 103–129.

Roberts, J. A., & Clement, A. (2007). Materialism and satisfaction with over-all quality of life and eight life domains. *Social Indicators Research, 82*(1), 79–92.

Robinson, J. P., & Martin, S. (2008). What do happy people do? *Social Indicators Research, 89*(3).

Rokach, A. (2004). The lonely and homeless: Causes and consequences. *Social Indicators Research, 69*(1), 37–50.

Rokach, A. (2006, September). Alienation and domestic abuse: How abused women cope with loneliness. *Social Indicators Research, 78*(2).

Rokach, A., & Orzecki, T. (2003, March). Coping with loneliness and drug use among young adults. *Social Indicators Research, 61*(3).

Ross, N. L. (2007). Engineering America's future. *Cosmos Bulletin, 60*(12), 22–23.

Royuela, V., Lopez-Tamayo, J., & Surinach, J. (2008, May). The institutional vs. the academic definition of the quality of work life. What is the focus of the European commission. *Social Indicators Research, 86*(3).

Rule, S. (2007, April). Religiosity and quality of life in South Africa. *Social Indicators Research, 81*(2).

Ryff, C. D., & Keyes, C. L. M. (1995). The structure of psychological well-being revisited. *Journal of Personality and Social Psychology, 69*(4), 719–727.

Sabates-Wheeler, R., Sabates, R., & Castaldo, A. (2008, June). Tracking poverty-migration linkages: Evidence from Ghana and Egypt. *Social Indicators Research, 87*(2).

Salmon, J. L. (2007, January 29–February 4). God's (Weight-Loss) plan. *The Washington Post National Weekly Edition*, p. 31.

Samli, A. C. (2008). Entrepreneurship, economic development and quality of life in third world countries. *Applied Research in Quality of Life, 3*(3).

Schimmack, U., Schupp, J., & Wagner, G. G. (2008, October). The influence environment and personality on the affective and cognitive component of subjective well-being. *Social Indicators Research, 89*(1).

Schmidt, S., & Power, M. (2006). Cross-cultural analyses of determinants of quality of life and mental health: Results from the EUROHIS study. *Social Indicators Research, 77*(1).

Schoch, R. (2006). *The secrets of happiness*. New York: Scribner.

Schwartz, S. H. (1992). Universals in the 'content and structure of values: Theoretical advances and empirical tests in 20 countries. In M. P. Zuna (Ed.). *Advances in Experimental Social Psychology* (Vol. 25, pp. 1–65), San Diego, CA: Academic Press.

Schwartz, S. H. (1994). Beyond individualism-collectivism: new cultural dimensions of values. In U. Kim, H. C. Triandis, C. Kagitchibasi, C. Choi, & G. Yon (Eds.), *Individualism and collectivism: Theory , method and applications* (pp. 85–102). Thousand Oaks, CA: Sage.

Seghiri, C., Desantis, G., & Tanturri, M. L. (2006). The richer, the happier? An empirical investigation in selected European countries. *Social Indicators Research, 79*(3).

Shenk, J. W. (2009, June). What makes us happy? *The Atlantic Monthly.*

Shew, D. M. (2007, Spring). Fighting extreme poverty, pathways. *Quarterly Journal of the Episcopal Diocese of Atlanta.*

Shu, X., & Zhu, Y. (2009, June) The quality of life in China. *Social Indicators Research, 92*(2).

Silva, L., Pais-Ribeiro, J., & Cardoso, H. (2008, June). Quality of life and general health perception in women with obesity. *Applied Research in Quality of Life, 3*(2).

Solzenberg, L., D'alessio, S. J., Rivers, J. E., & Newell, A. L. (2003, January). Measuring substance abuse treatment need among adults in Florida: A social indicators approach. *Social Indicators Research, 61*(1).

Sorokin, P. A. (1950). 'Love: Its aspects, production, transformation, and accumulation IV tentative considerations. Love energy. In P. A. Sorokin (Ed.) *Explorations in altruistic love and behavior.* Boston: The Beacon Press.

Surgy, M. J., Reilly, N. P., Wu, J., & Efraty, D. (2008). A work-life identity model of well-being: Towards a research agenda linking quality of work life (QOWL) programs with quality of life (QOL). *Applied Research in Quality of Life, 3*(3).

Suzuki, K. (2009). Are they frigid to the economic development? Reconsideration of the economic effect of subjective well-being. *Social Indicators Research, 92*(1).

Talbot, M. (2008, November 3). Red sex, Blue sex. *The New Yorker.*

Tan, S. J., Tambyah, S. K., & Kau, A. K. (2006). The influence of value orientations and demographics on quality of life perceptions: Evidence from a national survey of Singaporeans. *Social Indicators Research, 78*(1).

Teichmann, M., Murdvee, M., & Saks, K. (2006). Spiritual needs and quality of life in Estonia. *Social Indicators Research, 76*(1).

Tesch-Romer, C., Motel-Kingebiel, A., & Tomasik, M. J. (2008). Gender differences in subjective well-being: Comparing societies with respect to gender equality. *Social Indicators Research, 85*(2).

Texler, D. (2006). Extension. In H. J. Birx (ed.), *Encyclopedia of anthropology*. Thousand Oaks, CA: Sage.

Van Gundy, A. B. (1981). *Techniques of structured problem solving*. New York: Van Nostrand Renhold.

Veehhoven, R., & Hagerty, M. L. (2006). Rising happiness in nations, 1946–2004: A reply to Easterlin. *Social Indicators Research, 79*(3).

Veehhoven, R., & Hagerty, M. L. (2009). Well-being in nations and well-being of nations: Is there a conflict between individual and society? *Social Indicators Research, 91*(1).

Veenhoven, R., (1993). *Bibliography of Happiness*. Rotterdam: Erasmus University.

Vella-Brodrick, D. A., Park, N., & Peterson, C. (2009). Three ways to be happy: Pleasure, engagement and meaning – findings from Australian and U.S. samples. *Social Indicators Research, 90*(2).

Walton, D., Murray, S. J., & Thomas, J. A. (2008). Relationships between population density and the perceived quality of neighborhood. *Social Indicators Research, 89*(3).

Whyte, W. F. (1943). *Street corner society.* Chicago: University of Chicago Press.

Wilson, E. G. (2008). *Against happiness: In praise of melancholy.* New York: Farrar, Straus, Giroux.

Wisecup, A., Robinson, D. T., & Smith-Lovin, L. (2007). The sociology of emotions. In C. D. Bryant & D. L. Peck (Eds.), *21st century sociology.* Thousand Oaks, London, New Delhi: Sage Publications.

Wortham, R. A., & Wortham, C. B. (2007). Spiritual capital and the 'good life'. *Sociological Spectrum 27*(4), 439–452.

Yuan, A. S. (2008). Racial composition of neighborhood and emotional well-being. *Sociological Spectrum, 28*(1), 105–129.

Zahran, H. S., Kobau, R., Moriarty, D. G., Zack, M. M., Holt, J., & Donehoo, R. (2005). Health-Related Quality of Life Surveillance – United States, 1993–2002. *Morbidity and Mortality Weekly Report,* 54/no. SS-4. Atlanta: Centers for Disease Control and Prevention.

Zanner, R. M. (2002). What a wonderful world! In J. Howie (Ed.), *Ethical issues for a new millennium.* Carbondale and Edwardsville, IL: Southern Illinois University Press.

Zimmer, C., Dunn, K., & Kahn, J. (2006). Scientist of the year. *Discover, 27*(12), 35–37.

Zullig, K. J., Ward, R. M., & Horn, T. (2006). The association between perceived spirituality, religiosity, and life satisfaction: The mediating role of self-related health. *Social Indicators Research, 79*(2).

Index